This concise and practical book is designed for paediatricians and endocrinologists trained or in training, who see children with endocrine problems. All the endocrine glands are covered, and the author has distilled his vast experience and expertise in this area to provide hard-hitting, practical advice on the diagnosis, management, and treatment of the main endocrine disorders. It is not a heavily referenced tome but a monograph in the true sense of the word – a book in which an expert describes and discusses the area of his expertise for the benefit and interest of others. The volume is illustrated throughout and the text is also supplemented by many succinct and informative tables. The volume concludes with a short chapter on practical procedures, including endocrine tests, imaging, and drugs and doses.

A GUIDE TO THE PRACTICE OF PAEDIATRIC ENDOCRINOLOGY

A GUIDE TO THE PRACTICE OF PAEDIATRIC ENDOCRINOLOGY

C. G. D. BROOK, MA, MD(CANTAB), FRCP, DCH

Professor of Paediatric Endocrinology
University College London
Consultant Paediatrician
The Middlesex Hospital, London W1N 8AA, UK

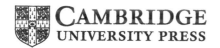

CAMBRIDGE
UNIVERSITY PRESS

CAMBRIDGE UNIVERSITY PRESS
Cambridge, New York, Melbourne, Madrid, Cape Town, Singapore, São Paulo

Cambridge University Press
The Edinburgh Building, Cambridge CB2 8RU, UK

Published in the United States of America by Cambridge University Press, New York

www.cambridge.org
Information on this title: www.cambridge.org/9780521431798

First published 1993
This digitally printed version (with corrections) 2007

A catalogue record for this publication is available from the British Library

Library of Congress Cataloguing in Publication data

Brook, C. G. D. (Charles Groves Darville)
A guide to the practice of paediatric endocrinology / C.G.D.
Brook
    p.   cm.
Includes index.
ISBN 0-521-43179-4 (hardback)
1. Pediatric endocrinology.   I. Title.
[DNLM: 1. Endocrine Diseases – in infancy and childhood.   WS330
B871g]
RJ418.B725   1993
618.92′4 – dc20
DNLM/DLC
for library of Congress   92-49015 CIP

ISBN 978-0-521-43179-8 hardback
ISBN 978-0-521-04677-0 paperback

Contents

Preface

In 1978 I published a small book about paediatric endocrinology. Since that time, there has been an amazing advance in many aspects of the practice of the discipline and some of my more loyal friends, Dr Stephen Herman in particular, have been kind enough to say that it is time for the subject to be brought up to date in a completely new book. This is it – and I thank Peter Silver and the Cambridge University Press for the opportunity to prepare it. Mary Sanders was extremely efficient in getting the book into print.

The Press told me that in a monograph 'an expert describes and discusses the area of his own expertise for the benefit and interest of others' which is what I have done. I hope that it will be useful to general paediatricians and endocrinologists. It encapsulates my view of the subject, which may be iconoclastic in places, and it is a practical book not a major work of critical analysis heavily referenced for the specialist in the field – I edit a much bigger volume for that purpose.

I would probably never have summoned the strength to set pen to paper in this venture were it not for the opportunity afforded to me to undertake a sabbatical exchange visit to the Royal Children's Hospital in Melbourne where I wrote the book. Dr John Court was generous enough to swap jobs, houses and cars for 5 months to enable this to happen and I am very grateful to him, to Cathy, my wife, for giving up her job and to our hospital and university colleagues in England and Australia for allowing us to exchange, and for their welcomes. I had a marvellous time; I hope that Dr Court enjoyed himself as much.

Over the years at The Middlesex I have been very happy, thanks to many people. I would like particularly to acknowledge the stimulation and support I have had from Peter Hindmarsh, Howard Jacobs, Antony Kurtz, Steve Semple, Jimmy Steele, Jeffrey O'Riordan, Sandra Ramsden and, most especially, Jane Pringle. I should also like to thank several generations of house physicians, registrars, research fellows, technicians and secretaries whose work has made possible what has been achieved. On this occasion, Emily Whitehead has been my secretary and has put up uncomplainingly with my importunities over the months: I am very grateful to her for her patient help.

C. G. D. Brook

August, 1992

1
Intersex

The first question a mother asks at delivery is the sex of her baby: when her question is met by anything but an unambiguous answer (Fig. 1.1), the consequences assume a lifelong importance.

Establishment of chromosomal sex occurs at the time of fertilization when the ovum is fertilized by a sperm bearing an X or Y chromosome. Since embryos carrying the Y chromosome develop as males, regardless of the number of X chromosomes, the conclusion is that the presence of the Y chromosome plays a critical role in switching on a complex process of male differentiation.

Sexual determination

Embryos of both sexes develop in a similar manner until 6–7 weeks of gestation, after which development diverges to result in male or female phenotype. In the presence of a Y chromosome, the undifferentiated gonad develops into a testis; in its absence it develops into an ovary but it can be extremely difficult histologically to determine which is which in the early stages of this process. The mechanism by which this occurs is still being debated.

The histocompatibility–Y antigen (H–Y antigen) was discovered when skin grafts from male to female mice were rejected but no reaction was documented from females to males or between the same sex. As the gene for the H–Y antigen was located on the Y chromosome, it was assumed to be the sex-determining gene but this hypothesis was not adequate to explain why a human XX male was described with negative H–Y antigen nor a XY female with positive H–Y antigen status.

DNA hybridization using Y specific probes in XX males and XY females have yielded separate genetic loci for the H–Y antigen and the sex

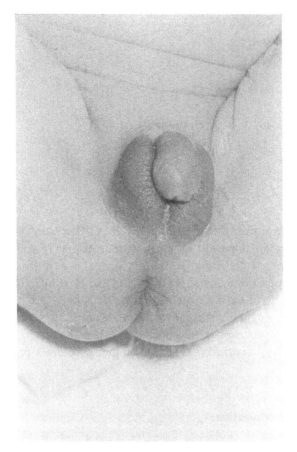

Fig. 1.1. Ambiguous genitalia – little boy or little girl?

determining region on the Y chromosome (SRY), formerly called the testicular determining factor (TDF). The SRY maps to the tip of the short arm of the Y chromosome and the gene controlling H–Y antigen maps to the long arm. There are probably also autosomal determinants of sexual determination in man and it is possible that the autosomal genes produce a precursor substance in embryos of both sexes which is transformed by SRY in the male to a testicular inducing antigen. It is possible that this antigen may have a part to play in spermatogenesis. Despite convincing evidence for SRY as the testis inducer, most XX true hermaphrodites and 20 % of XX males have no Y chromosome sequences, so the mystery of male sexual determination remains unsolved.

What matters in the general clinical practice of the real world is that a Y chromosome is required for testes to be present in the fetus.

Sexual differentiation

Differentiation of gonads

The primitive gonad develops from the blastemal mass and primordial germ cells which migrate from the posterior endoderm of the yolk sac. In the presence of a Y chromosome, primitive seminiferous tubules form in the centre of the gonad. Germ cells are incorporated and nurtured by the surrounding Sertoli cells. Fetal Leydig cells differentiate from the mesenchyme and produce testosterone in response to stimulation by placental human chorionic gonadotrophin (HCG) and later by fetal pituitary LH.

In the absence of a Y chromosome, the undifferentiated gonad has an inherent tendency to develop as an ovary. The germ cells undergo mitotic and meiotic divisions and develop as oocytes. These become enveloped by a layer of granulosa cells and are known as primordial follicles. The formation of these reaches a maximum of 7 million or thereabouts during the 20th to 25th weeks of gestation and they then become progressively atretic over the rest of life (Fig. 1.2). With the surge of fetal pituitary FSH, the first primary follicles are formed.

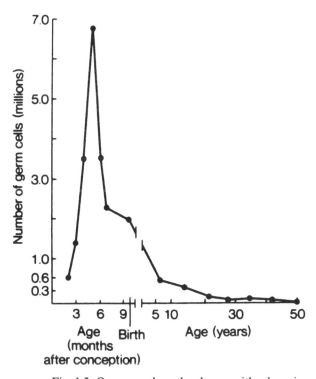

Fig. 1.2. Ovum number; the change with advancing years.

Differentiation of genital ducts

Around the fourth week of gestation the Wolffian ducts develop and open into the cloaca. The Müllerian ducts develop slightly later and, by the eighth week, both ducts are complete. The presence of the fetal testis determines the further direction of genital duct differentiation in the male (Fig. 1.3).

Differentiation of the Wolffian ducts into epididymis, vas deferens and seminal vesicles requires high local concentrations of testosterone from the fetal Leydig cells and the presence of androgen receptors to which testosterone can bind directly. This contrasts with the development of the external genitalia which requires the conversion of testosterone to dihydrotestosterone by the enzyme 5-α reductase.

The fetal testis has another quite separate role through the local (paracrine) secretion of a glycoprotein, called antimüllerian hormone (AMH), by the Sertoli cells of the seminiferous tubules. This causes regression of the Müllerian ducts from 9–11 weeks by acting on cell surface receptors on the underlying mesenchyme rather than on the epithelium of the ducts.

AMH has other important roles. First, it inhibits intratesticular aromatase, thus preventing the conversion of testosterone to estradiol.

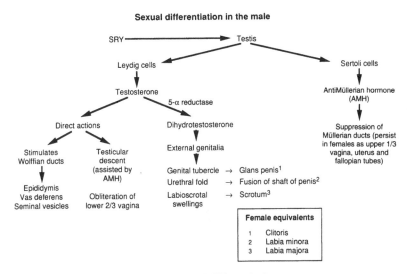

Fig. 1.3. The process of sexual differentiation.

Secondly, it has an as-yet not clearly defined role in promoting descent of the testis. Thirdly, it prevents progression of germ cells beyond meiosis so that spermatogenesis can only proceed when local concentrations of AMH decline, as they do before and during puberty.

In patients with true hermaphroditism, in whom both ovary and testis are present, the regression of Müllerian ducts is most marked on the side of the testis. In patients with androgen insensitivity, müllerian derivatives are absent because of AMH secretion and wolffian derivatives are absent because of androgen resistance.

In females, the wolffian ducts disappear. The upper parts of the müllerian ducts develop into the fallopian tubes, the middle parts into the uterus and the lower parts into the upper one third of the vagina. This development occurs independently of the presence or absence of the ovaries and exposure to androgens does not affect it.

Differentiation of external genitalia

The external genitalia develop from the genital tubercle, the urogenital groove, which is bounded by paired urethral folds and labioscrotal swellings, and the urogenital sinus into which both müllerian and wolffian systems open.

In the male, the development of the external genitalia is dependent upon the presence of 5α dihydrotestosterone, which is derived from the conversion of testosterone by the enzyme 5α reductase, which is found in high concentration in these tissues. The genital tubercle becomes the glans penis and the fusion of the urethral folds and groove form the shaft of the penis. The labioscrotal swellings fuse and enlarge to become the scrotum into which the testes descend. AMH is responsible for descent of the testes to the inguinal region from where testosterone takes over, carrying the wolffian duct derivatives with the testes into the scrotum. The latest evidence is that testosterone masculinizes the genito-femoral nerve and promotes the elaboration of calcitonin gene related peptide (CGRP), a 37 amino acid protein, which causes gubernacular contraction.

In the female, the genital tubercle becomes the clitoris, the labioscrotal swellings the labia majora and the urethral folds the labia minora. The urogenital sinus forms the lower two thirds of the vagina.

Hormonal control

Although fetal pituitary gonadotrophin secretion may start as early as the fifth week of gestation, it does not contribute greatly to wolffian duct differentiation, the major stimulus to the fetal leydig cells being placental HCG. After the critical period of sex differentiation, continued growth of the fetal testis is dependent on pituitary gonadotrophins which reach a peak around 20 weeks and stimulate the testes to produce concentrations of testosterone which are similar to adult male values. Placental HCG and fetal LH act together to produce normal growth of the penis and scrotum and descent of the testes. This is why micropenis and bilateral cryptorchidism are characteristic of congenital gonadotrophin deficiency.

The placenta is the overwhelming source of estrogen in the female fetus but fetal FSH is important for growth and maintenance of folliculogenesis.

After birth, the removal of the negative feedback of placental hormones provokes a surge of gonadotrophin secretion which results in high concentrations of LH and FSH in the newborn period. This is partly due also to a fourfold increase in sex hormone binding globulin levels after birth. During the first six years of life, gonadotrophin levels fall progressively, and the hypothalamo-pituitary–gonadal axis becomes relatively quiescent in middle childhood. Nevertheless, the system is not inactive: occasional episodic secretion of LH and FSH can be seen in 24 h profiles of hormone concentrations in young children and a lack of gonadal response will provoke a rise in concentrations of LH and FSH, as seen in agonadal boys or girls.

Abnormal sexual development

Disorders of intersex have traditionally been classified into three main categories, each given a rather grand name. Patients with a 46XX karyotype with normal ovaries and female internal genitalia, but with varying degrees of external virilization, have been called female pseudohermaphrodites. Patients with a 46XY karyotype, whose gonads are testes, but whose genital ducts, external genitalia or both are inadequately masculinised, have been called male pseudohermaphrodites. Hermaphrodites have tissue of both testicular and ovarian origin. I do not think that the first two terms are helpful to the management of the clinical problem of intersex and propose to abandon them.

Virilized females

The degree of virilization of the external genitalia of a female fetus depends on the concentration of androgen to which the fetus is exposed and on the time in gestation when the exposure takes place. The degree can be usefully categorized according to the Prader stage (Fig 1.4). Exposure to androgens

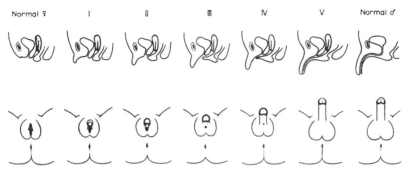

Fig. 1.4. Appearance of external genitalia from normal female to male with Prader stages I–V of genital ambiguity. (*Helv. Paediatr. Acta* (1954) **9**, 231–48)

in the second trimester, when the vagina has already differentiated from the urogenital sinus, leads only to clitoral hypertrophy. Earlier exposure results in retention of the urogenital sinus and labioscrotal fusion. Müllerian duct differentiation proceeds normally even in the presence of the most severe virilization; a fetus without a testis virtually always develops a uterus, although the syndrome of an embryonal failure of uterine development in the presence of normal ovarian function does occur.

The causes of virilization are shown in Table 1.1. The commonest are the forms of congenital adrenal hyperplasia, which will be discussed in detail in Chapter 5 (page 109). Exposure to androgens of maternal origin is less

Table 1.1. *Causes of virilization*

Virilization by androgens of fetal origin
Congenital adrenal hyperplasia
Persistent fetal adrenocortical steroids
Virilization by androgens of maternal origin
Iatrogenic – anabolic steroids
testosterone
progestagens
danazol
Tumours of ovary or adrenal glands
Congenital adrenal hyperplasia
Dysmorphic syndromes, e.g. Seckel, Zellweger, Beckwith
Local abnormalities, such as neurofibromatosis
lipoma
hemangioma
Idiopathic

common; these may arise from neoplastic change in the ovary or adrenal or, more likely, be ingested by the mother in the form of progestagens (which are associated with the causation of hypospadias), danazol, a derivative of ethinyl testosterone used for the treatment of endometriosis, and anabolic steroids such as those abused by athletes. A mother with congenital adrenal hyperplasia may become pregnant if her condition is properly treated and the treatment has to be especially monitored during the pregnancy if the fetus is not to become virilized.

Ambiguity of the genitalia, particularly clitoral hypertrophy, is associated with some rare dysmorphic syndromes. Clitoral hypertrophy can also be seen in the very premature infant in whom the fetal adrenal cortex produces large amounts of a weak androgen, dehydroepiandrosterone sulphate (DHEAS), in the newborn nursery. The clitoral hypertrophy which results usually disappears towards what would have been term and/or becomes less obvious as fat accumulates in the labia, but it sometimes persists into childhood and may need surgical correction. Sometimes the virilization of a female fetus defies explanation even after exhaustive tests and only time may reveal its cause.

Inadequately masculinized males

Incomplete masculinization of the genital ducts and external genitalia may result in a clinical appearance ranging from the apparently normal female to a male with hypospadias and/or cryptorchidism. With the exception of the persistent Müllerian duct syndrome, males with functional testicular tissue lose Müllerian duct structures.

Poor masculinization (Table 1.2) may result from LH deficiency, Leydig cell hypoplasia, disorders of testosterone biosynthesis and abnormalities of the effects of testosterone in the peripheral tissues. The pathway of testosterone biosynthesis is shown in Fig. 1.5 together with estrogen conversion.

As already indicated, testosterone has to be converted in the external genitalia to dihydrotesterone by 5α-reductase to have its effect in fetal life. When this enzyme is absent, a curious syndrome develops. The infant has ambiguous genitalia (Fig. 1.6) but the testes are present in the labioscrotal folds because they descend under the direct influence of testosterone with the co-action of AMH. Testosterone (and not DHT) is responsible for male pubertal development, so these patients apparently 'change sex' in the teenage years when the clitoris grows under the influence of LH-stimulated testosterone production.

Table 1.2. *Causes of inadequate masculinization*

Leydig cell agenesis or hypoplasia
LH deficiency
Inborn errors of testosterone biosynthesis
    Affecting testes and adrenal glands
        Cholesterol side chain cleavage deficiency
        3β-hydroxysteroid dehydrogenase deficiency
        17α-hydroxylase deficiency
    Affecting testes
        17,20-lyase deficiency
        17β-hydroxysteroid dehydrogenase deficiency
Defect in target tissues
    Defect in testosterone metabolism
        5α-reductase deficiency
    Androgen receptor and postreceptor defects
Persistent Müllerian duct syndrome
    AMH deficiency
Associated with dysmorphic syndromes
    e.g. Smith–Lemli–Opitz, Dubowitz, Aniridia–Wilms, etc.

End organ resistance to androgen action may be due to quantitative or qualitative defects in the receptors, defects in intracellular transport of receptor generated proteins, defects in activation of nuclear binding sites, in transcription or in translation of the message. These defects are inherited in a sex-linked recessive manner.

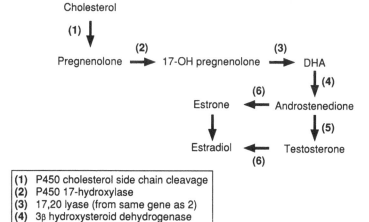

Fig. 1.5. Pathway of testosterone biosynthesis and estrogen conversion.

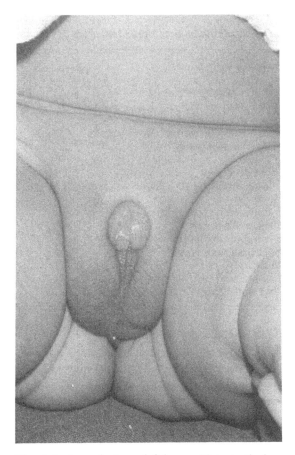

Fig. 1.6. 5α reductase deficiency. Note testicular swelling in right labioscrotal fold.

When there is complete androgen insensitivity, the genitalia remain female but the müllerian structures are lost, resulting in a short vagina. Breast development occurs secondary to estrogen production without testosterone opposition at puberty but there is no pubic or axillary hair growth; the syndrome thus used to be called testicular feminization. There are many degrees of androgen insensitivity so that patients may have a normal female appearance or may have degrees of virilization, perineo-scrotal hypospadias or cryptorchidism. The whole picture becomes still more complicated (and distressing) when sex steroids are secreted at the time of puberty.

Failure of the Sertoli cells to secrete AMH or failure of the müllerian ducts to respond to it results in a phenotypically normal male who has normal female internal genitalia (uterus and fallopian tubes) as well as normal male structures. Most patients with this condition probably go undetected unless they develop a hernia, which may contain the uterus. The surgeon confronted with this situation must not be tempted to remove the uterus, the presence of which will do the patient no harm, because the vas usually runs through the myometrium; hysterectomy thus renders the patient sterile. Whether fertility is the rule in these patients is not known because normal males do not get examined with this problem in mind. Some patients do, however, come to light in infertility clinics with this diagnosis.

Disorders of gonadal differentiation

Because of the dual role of the fetal testis, all combinations of abnormality of the external and internal genitalia can occur. This applies particularly to patients with dysgenetic gonads which have varying degrees of functional capability.

Patients with pure gonadal dysgenesis most frequently have XY or XO karyotypes but chromosomal mosaicism is probably the rule rather than the exception in the latter (see discussion of the Turner syndrome). These patients present as females with primary amenorrhoea.

Patients with mixed gonadal dysgenesis typically have a testis palpable either in the inguinal region or the scrotum with perineal hypospadias. Wolffian structures and absent müllerian structures are found ipsilateral to the testis. On the other side, a streak gonad is found with müllerian structures and absent wolffian development.

More common are boys with functional anorchia, so called 'vanishing testes syndrome', who present with normal male genitalia and bilateral cryptorchidism. Such patients must have had testicular function in the fetal period to differentiate as males and not have a uterus, but no functioning testes can be shown. They need help at puberty.

True hermaphrodites have well-developed ovarian and testicular tissues in either the same or opposite gonads. A testis on one side, and ovary on the other, constitutes about 30% of patients, bilateral ovotestes about 20%, and the remainder have an ovotestis on one side and a normal testis or ovary on the other. The wolffian and müllerian duct development follows the lead of the ipsilateral gonad. External genitalia may be ambiguous but the condition can present with a hernia containing a gonad or a müllerian derivative or at puberty when anything can happen. Menstruation occurs in 50% of female hermaphrodites, and pregnancy and childbirth have been documented. The karyotype may be XX, XY or XX/XY.

Although most XX males have a male phenotype, ambiguous genitalia have been reported in some patients.

Diagnosis, management and treatment

The first rule is not to panic when confronted with an infant with ambiguous genitalia. It is most important to take time to get the diagnosis right and to assign a sex of rearing after appropriate professional consultation and discussion with the parents of the child, who are usually devastated by the enormity of the problem. The people to consult will include a gynaecologist, urologist and possibly a psychiatrist or psychotherapist. The parents should be assured as far as possible that there will be a clear outcome, in the decision about which their opinions are extremely important, but they should be warned that the decision-making process takes time, sometimes quite a lot of time, to achieve a diagnosis. It does not usually take as long to make a plan of how to proceed.

The birth should not be registered until the sex of rearing has been decided; altering the Register if the sex of the child has been wrongly registered is a difficult legal process while delaying registration is easy. Allied to this issue is that of naming the child. Obviously this is something which every parent longs to do but I believe that it is better to help the parents restrain this intention until the sex of rearing has been decided with their agreement. They can then choose an unambiguously male or female name which will help bonding with the child in a manner appropriate for sex. I have not found that the choice of an ambiguous name (e.g.Francis or Frances, Lesley or Leslie) for a baby with this difficult problem to be in anybody's interest, regardless of what may appear to be its superficial attraction.

The second rule is not to jump to conclusions. It is not possible to make a diagnosis from the phenotypic appearance of the infant with ambiguous genitalia, and diagnostic procedures must, therefore, be followed in an orderly fashion in all cases to establish a line of management.

How to proceed

A careful history and examination of the mother may be instructive if she shows signs of virilization and/or admits to ingestion of drugs or medications. Special attention should be paid to parental consanguinity

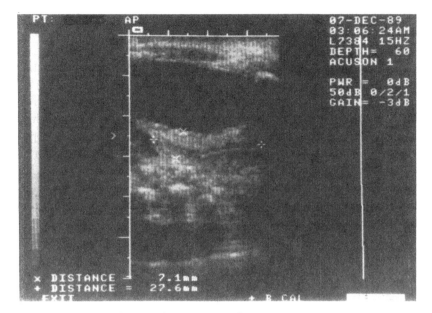

Fig. 1.7. Ultrasound appearance of neonatal uterus. Note endometrial echo from the effect of maternal estrogen.

and family history of primary amenorrhoea, infertility, late puberty and unexplained neonatal deaths in siblings or relatives.

Physical examination of the baby should include a search for other congenital abnormalities and dysmorphic features. It may reveal the presence of testes which will greatly assist the line of thought. The position of the urethral meatus is less helpful.

The first investigation of major importance is pelvic ultrasonography. In the practice of paediatric endocrinology this non-invasive technique is invaluable. But it is not easy, and especially not in the newborn, in whom it is a matter of patience to coincide an examination with the occurrence of a full bladder. We have the mother and baby together in our ultrasound department and examine the latter at regular intervals during a (hopefully breast) feed until it is possible to decide whether or not a uterus is present. The dimensions of the newborn uterus are, of course, increased by maternal estrogen so this examination is not as difficult as it becomes later in the infantile period (Fig. 1.7).

If a uterus is present, the baby is almost certainly a virilized female, in which case congenital adrenal hyperplasia (CAH) becomes much the most likely diagnosis; if it is absent, the diagnosis is likely to be more difficult to establish. It is very difficult to tell with certainty an ovary from a testis on ultrasound examination of the newborn but, in the absence of a uterus, gonadal structures can be presumed to be testes and the recording of their position is helpful.

An experienced ultrasonographer can visualize much of the urogenital system so, particularly in the absence of a uterus, it may be possible to delineate the urethra and its possible connections to a urogenital sinus. At The Middlesex, we rarely find it necessary to resort to radiographic contrast studies, such as urethrograms or vaginograms, nor to laparoscopy or indeed laparotomy to define internal structures, but we are particularly fortunate in the quality of our ultrasound service. Travel has shown me that not all colleagues are so fortunate and the scale of the structures to be imaged daunts many operators skilled in the practice of ultrasound in paediatric and adult patients. Perseverance is the key to success.

Blood tests

Appropriate samples should be taken for:

- Karyotype
- Electrolytes, urea and creatinine
- 17α-hydroxyprogesterone, testosterone, androstenedione, DHT and DHEA
- LH, FSH
- ACTH, plasma renin activity, aldosterone and other hormones which may be needed later.
- Two further samples are needed. The first, for hormone assay, should be separated and stored for possible future use. From the second DNA should be extracted and stored for future analysis leading to genetic counselling, antenatal diagnosis and possible therapy in future pregnancies.

Urine tests

A 24 h collection of urine should be made for analysis of steroid excretion profile.

Stimulation tests

It may be necessary to stimulate potential testicular tissue in cases of inadequate masculinization with HCG and to measure the steroids secreted. This is not usually necessary because LH levels are generally high in the newborn period but the procedure may clarify a difficult situation, such as 5α-reductase deficiency, by highlighting the altered ratio of testosterone to dihydrotestosterone produced in response to stimulation.

Stimulation with ACTH is also sometimes useful but not until the baseline investigations have been assessed.

Invasive tests

Invasive radiological and pelvic examinations are rarely required. In cases of potential androgen insensitivity, it is necessary to take samples of sex sensitive (genital) skin for the culture of fibroblasts and assessment of androgen receptor mechanisms.

Gender assignment

A decision on the sex of rearing should be reached as soon as possible. This should be based mainly on the possibility of achieving unambiguous and functionally normal external genitalia and reproductive capability where possible through surgery, hormonal therapy or both. The karyotype is not important in making this decision but the presence of a uterus is very relevant in view of the prospects for embryo transfer.

When considering the male gender, the size of the penis is important but not as important as its potential to grow. A disaster could arise if a patient was brought up in the male gender role and it was then found impossible adequately to masculinize him at puberty because of androgen insensitivity. Fortunately, this situation can be tested in the newborn period by giving three injections of testosterone 25 mg at monthly intervals and observing the effect on the size of the phallus. I find clinical photography to be very helpful in making an objective assessment.

Infants with 5α-reductase deficiency with an adequate phallus should be raised as males and correction of the external genitalia (removal of chordee, meatoplasty, etc) should be done early. If a late diagnosis has been made, and the sex of rearing has been female, consideration should be given to cliteroplasty and orchidectomy rather than a sex role change at the onset of puberty. The induction of breast development should not be difficult (see Chapter 10, page 171) and this course may be followed in other cases where a change in gender may be more upsetting than a continuation of the perceived gender, such as a case of 17β-hydroxysteroid dehydrogenase deficiency who may masculinize at puberty through gonadotrophin stimulation of the testes. A patient such as this, who is unable to make intratesticular testosterone will not achieve normal spermatogenesis, so, even though she may not have a uterus, it may be preferable to stay in the female role.

Patients with CAH need careful long-term management (see Chapter 5, page 109). In the newborn period, care should be taken to avoid hypoglycemia and a careful watch should be kept on the electrolyte concentrations to diagnose and treat a salt-losing state before it become a crisis. A rising serum potassium concentration and/or weight loss are the best guides to this.

The place of surgery

The importance of early reconstructive surgery needs emphasis because it helps to allay lingering doubts the parents may have regarding the sex of their child, and helps avoid rejection by family and friends alike. The issue of bonding is important in babies with intersex: everything possible must be organized to keep mother and baby closely attached while the diagnostic and therapeutic manoeuvres are being endured. Breast feeding is a good way to ensure this.

Clitoral reduction, separation of labia and limited vaginoplasty should be undertaken between three and six months of age, although more extensive vaginal operations may have to wait until the child is somewhat older (but preschool) and may well have to be revised around the pubertal years, especially when the patient desires sexual intercourse. There is something of a problem here in timing: vaginal stretching requires regular use of a dilator or regular intercourse to prevent restenosis. There is no point in starting treatment too early but, on the other hand, the patient's desire for the possibility of intercourse must be respected but without coercion in that direction. Having continuous care for the child from the same gynaecologist throughout is probably the best answer.

For those who are assigned the male role, there may be need for a series of operations stretching over a number of years, The aim should certainly be to have the patient urinating standing up by the time he goes to school but the need for ongoing psychological support is considerable and too frequently overlooked.

Gonadectomy

Patients with dysgenetic or non-functional gonads, especially those with Y-bearing cell lines (males with functional anorchia, girls with gonadal dysgenesis and hermaphrodites), have an increased risk of malignant change in the gonad. This risk is very small before puberty and rises to about 30% of neoplastic change in situ by the fourth decade. With ultrasound monitoring, gonadectomy can and, in my opinion, should be delayed until after puberty has been completed in patients with total androgen insensitivity because it gives the possibility for a 'natural' puberty. In patients with partial androgen insensitivity, and in those with deficient testosterone biosynthesis who are assigned to the female gender, it is best to remove the testes prepubertally to prevent virilization at puberty. Patients should receive appropriate pubertal induction and maintenance therapy.

Psychological support

Before gender assignment, a simple explanation of the physiology of sexual differentiation with anatomical drawings helps understanding of the situation and defuses the idea that adult men and women are actually as different as they may seem. However speed and competence go a long way to helping the acceptance of the baby and the bonding process.

Sexual identity becomes firmly established in children aged 3–4 years but the acceptance of a 'change of sex' at puberty in communities where 5α-reductase deficiency is common emphasizes that gender is not immutable. It is obvious, however, that reassignment of sex after the newborn period should not be undertaken lightly, and decisions of this nature require intensive support for the family.

In families where children with ambiguous genitalia have been managed with knowledge, experience and expedition, the psychological support required by the parents and children during childhood is usually minimal. Either, or both, may require psychotherapeutic help before, during and after puberty. For this reason, if for no other, these patients do best if managed in centres used to dealing with the problem. The children also cope better later if they are enabled to share all knowledge about diagnosis and prognosis as early as possible. I do not think that it is necessary for a girl to be burdened with the knowledge that she has a Y-bearing cell line but the earlier she gets used to the idea that she will have difficulty in conceiving or carrying a child, the easier acceptance of this unpleasant reality becomes for her in adolescence. It is not a good idea to shield her from the truth, as any infertile woman will confirm.

2
Growth

Normal growth and its endocrine control

Growth begins at conception and reaches a peak in terms of height velocity during the second trimester, when the crown-heel rate attains a speed of 2 cm/week, the fastest the individual will ever grow. After that peak has been achieved, the velocity falls to around 5 mm/week at term. The increment in the first year of postnatal life is about 25 cm so that fetal and early postnatal growth account for nearly half of all the growth in adult length.

This broad brush summary conceals a wealth of ignorance of detail about growth at a critical time. Fast dividing cells are especially susceptible to adverse environmental circumstances and yet we know next to nothing about the complexity of factors which must govern the growth process at this critical time. This is clearly demonstrated by our inability to influence, or rather to correct, abnormal growth in utero and by our poor showing in attaining normal growth rates of premature infants in the newborn nursery.

Postnatal growth

The human growth curve has never been better exemplified than by that most famous of curves, the growth in length of the son of Count Philibert Gueneau de Montbeillard between 1759 and 1777 (Fig. 2.1). The upper panel of this Figure, the distance chart, shows the length as measured at 6-monthly intervals; the lower panel, the velocity chart, shows the annual increments plotted against the chronological age at the mid-points of each whole year.

From these charts it is easy to see the tripartite nature of human growth.

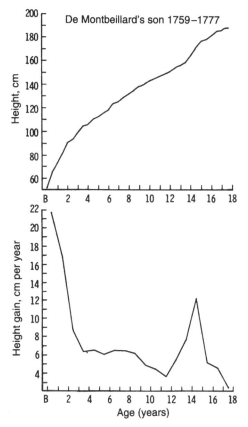

Fig. 2.1. Growth of the son of Count de Montbeillard. Upper panel: distance chart. Lower panel: velocity chart.

There is a rapid and rapidly decelerating phase of growth in infancy, a steady and slowly decelerating phase of growth in childhood, which is broken by the mid-childhood growth spurt between ages 5 and 9 (clearly seen in the velocity chart), and a growth spurt at puberty with a take-off in this boy in the 12th year of life. The understanding of the controlling mechanisms of these three (four) phases of growth and how they interact illumines the clinical practice of paediatrics (Fig. 2.2*a*).

Infantile growth

From conception and into the first year of life, the growth process is almost entirely dependent upon nutrition. Children with anencephaly, growth hormone deficiency due to deletion of the growth hormone gene or congenital hypothyroidism have a virtually normal body length at birth.

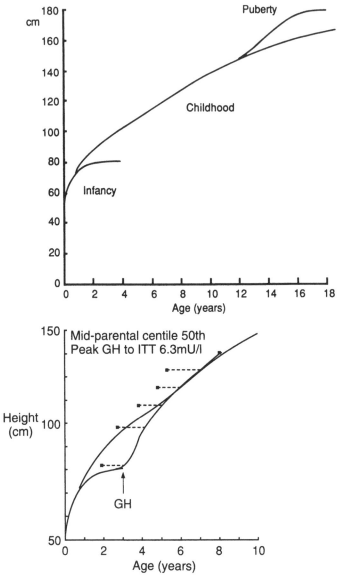

Fig. 2.2. (*a*) Infantile, childhood and puberty 50th centile values (after Karlberg). (*b*) Growth at a normal rate on the infantile curve of a child with GH insufficiency and the take-off with GH treatment.

The effects of intrauterine malnutrition are obvious in the delivery suite and of postnatal starvation obvious in the toll of disaster in Third World food shortages. The effects of calorie excess in utero are equally obvious in the infant of the diabetic mother, who is large as well as fat as a result of excessive glucose and insulin in utero, and in the infant fed excessively who becomes tall as well as fat. These facts, so obvious in animal husbandry, seem to be overlooked by physicians.

Childhood growth

Towards the end of the first year of postnatal life, a child with an isolated insufficiency of growth hormone secretion begins apparently to fail to thrive; in fact, as Fig. 2.2*b* shows, he tends to follow the centile curves for infantile growth derived mathematically by Dr Johann Karlberg entirely independently of any notion of causation from anthropometric data of children measured in Goteborg, Sweden over the years. Growth hormone receptors do not become detectable in the human infant until 200 days of postnatal life and this finding accords well with clinical observation, although more profound hormonal deficits may present earlier.

The timing of the take-off of the childhood curves from the infancy curves has important, but little appreciated, clinical consequences in individual children. The importance of timing has long been appreciated in the timing of the take-off of pubertal growth from the childhood curves, since it accounts for the difference in height between adult men and women. A late take-off of childhood growth has been documented, for example, in less affluent groups in Pakistan and this means that the children lose some height in infancy which they will probably never regain. The same can also apply to individual children seen in clinical paediatric practice in developed countries.

The growth rate of boys and girls is virtually identical during the childhood years and is related in an asymptotic manner to the amount of growth hormone they secrete (Fig. 2.3). This figure was compiled from the study of 50 short prepubertal children growing with a very wide range of velocities and a correspondingly wide range of peak amplitudes of growth hormone concentration.

The calculated asymptote B corresponds very closely to the growth rate observed in children with growth hormone deficiency secondary to deletion of the growth hormone gene. The asymptote A approximates a height velocity standard deviation score (Z-score) of zero in this group of children, which included a few short normal children growing normally along a low height centile. In the presence of a greater quantity of

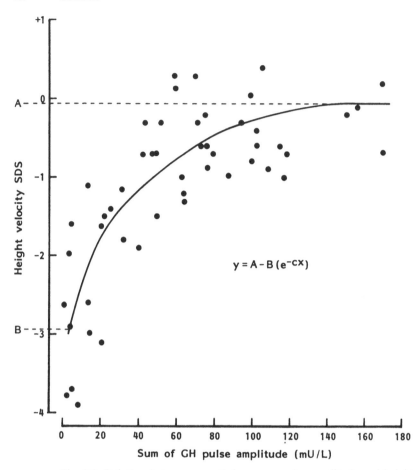

Fig. 2.3. Relation between growth hormone pulse amplitude and height velocity standard deviation score in 50 short prepubertal children (after Hindmarsh *et al.*, *Clin. Endocrinol.* (1987) **27**, 581–91).

endogenous growth hormone, as seen in tall children, the line must enter the positive range: tall children become and remain tall and become tall adults only by growing at a rate consistently slightly greater than that of their short peers. If the upper asymptote were not to enter the positive range, tall people in general, and pituitary giants in particular would not exist.

The experience of using first pituitary growth hormone and now biosynthetic growth hormone in unlimited amounts in clinical practice amply confirms the primacy of growth hormone as the controlling influence on childhood growth.

Mid-childhood growth spurt

Around the age of 6–8 years, boys and girls have an increase in the rate of growth. It is difficult to detect this in any study which is not purely longitudinal but it is well demonstrated in Fig. 2.1*b*.

The cause of this increase in growth rate is not well established but it coincides with the differentiation of the zona reticularis in the adrenal cortex and the detection of secretion of adrenal androgens, which can be marked in some children by the appearance of pubic and sometimes also axillary hair and by the secretion of apocrine axillary sweat. Adrenal androgens, which are ACTH stimulable and dexamethasone suppressible, could clearly influence growth rate and it is my belief that the onset of their secretion is the cause of the mid-childhood growth spurt. The loss of this spurt has serious clinical concomitants in the poor growth of, for example, asthmatic children, particularly if they are treated with steroid medications.

Pubertal growth

During childhood there are intermittent bursts of pulsatile gonadotrophin secretion (see Chapter 3, page 55) which eventually result in sufficient sex steroid secretion to become manifest as the secondary sexual characteristics. As soon as there is sufficient estradiol circulating to be manifest as breast development in a girl, the amplitude of pulsatile growth hormone secretion increases and growth velocity rises. In a boy of the same age, the growth velocity continues at a childhood rate (approximately 5 cm/year) for a further two years before the concentration of testosterone is sufficient to make an anabolic contribution in its own right and increase the amplitude of pulsatile growth hormone secretion, probably through aromatization to estradiol in the hypothalamo-pituitary axis. The growth rate then increases sharply to a peak which is somewhat greater than that of the girl (Fig. 2.4).

The delay in take-off on a distance curve which is still rising accounts for a final difference in adult heights of men and women of 10 cm. A further 5 cm is gained by boys through the magnitude of the peak height velocity, but 2.4 cm of this gain is lost by a boy stopping growing more quickly than a girl after the peak height velocity of adolescence has been reached. Thus, although the take-off differs by 2 years, the cessation of growth occurs only one year later in boys than in girls.

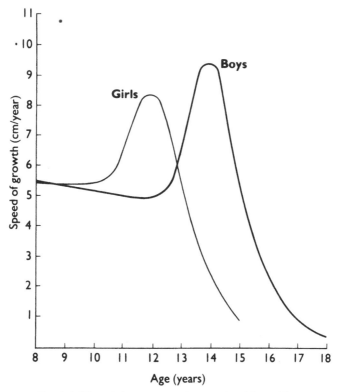

Fig. 2.4. The adolescent growth spurt in girls and boys

Cessation of growth

It is loosely correct to say that growth stops when the epiphyses fuse but what makes them actually do so is far from clear. It clearly has to do with sex steroids but an agonadal patient will stop growing, even though his epiphyses have not fused. From a clinical point of view it is important to recognize that the body stops growing from the feet upwards. The bones of the foot fuse, then the long bones and then the spine – hence the long-legged look of the adolescent. The iliac apophyses (Fig. 2.5) give a good guide to how much spinal growth is yet to come.

The larynx and face continue to grow after other growth has stopped but the description of this part of growth is much less complete than the earlier phases.

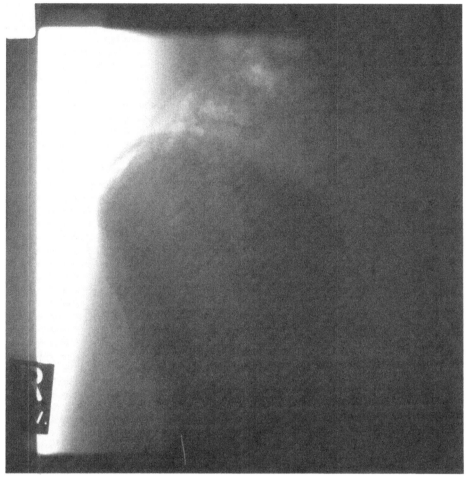

Fig. 2.5. Appearance of the iliac apophyses

Growth assessment

The essential tools of the trade are a device to measure standing and sitting heights in children and adults and lengths in babies, a skinfold caliper, orchidometer, tape measure, bone age assessment book and access to standard values, usually presented as charts. Weighing scales and anthropometer to measure girdle widths and limb lengths are optional extras. Using these tools is not difficult but data worth gathering need to be measured reliably and repeatably. Only the person who will be certainly be present on the next occasion the patient will attend should perform the measurements. It is quite possible for this person to be a physician, nurse,

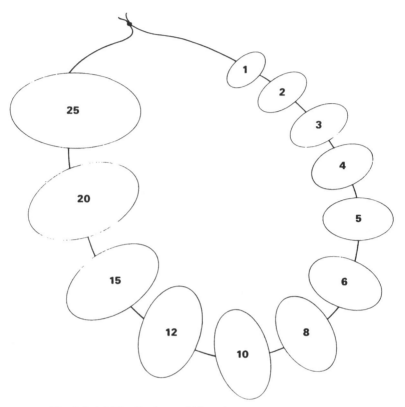

Fig. 2.6. (*a*) The Prader orchidometer.

secretary, receptionist or volunteer but it must always be the *same* person using the same technique time and again.

Instruments

The best anthropometric equipment (stadiometer for measuring height, sitting height table, infant measuring tables, etc) is available from Holtain Ltd, Crosswell, Crymych, Dyfed SA41 3UF, UK (Tel. 44–23–979–656, Fax 44–23–979–453). Standard charts are usually available appropriate for the local population. A very useful compilation of UK standards may be found in Buckler, JMH (1979), A reference manual of growth and development, Blackwell Scientific Publications, Oxford (ISBN 0–632–00185–2). UK Charts are available from Castlemead Publications, 12 Little Mundells, Welwyn Garden City, Herts AL7 1EW, UK (Tel. 44–707–320220, Fax 44–707–331012).

The technique of measuring lengths lying, standing or sitting is first to

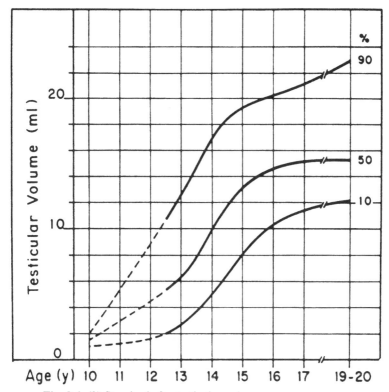

Fig. 2.6. (*b*) Standards for testicular volume.

ensure that the head is held in a standard position with the outer canthus of the eye in the same horizontal plane as the external auditory meatus. The maximum length is then obtained by exerting gentle traction on the mastoid processes with audible encouragement to be as straight as possible: 'Take a deep breath, breathe out, relax'. The measurement is then recorded from the scale, which should be checked for accuracy at the start of each clinic session.

I use measurements of sitting height for two purposes, first to assess body proportions and, secondly, to give a check on my measurement of stature. Measuring sitting height requires some sort of box of known height upon which the patient sits under the height scale. A custom made sitting height table is ideal but not essential. The height of the box is determined either by using the scale of the stadiometer or by using the standard rule, which is supplied to check accuracy of the counter, and primary school mathematics.

I find it useful to record triceps and subscapular skinfold thicknesses, but

Table 2.1. *Fractions of growth elapsed for a given skeletal age*

Skeletal age	Boys	Girls
6.0	67.0%	72%
7.0	69.5	75.7
8.0	72.3	79.0
9.0	75.2	82.7
10.0	78.4	86.2
11.0	80.4	90.6
12.0	83.4	92.2
13.0	87.6	95.8
14.0	92.7	98.0
15.0	96.8	99.0
16.0	98.2	99.6
17.0	99.1	99.9
18.0	99.6	100.0

Bayley and Pinneau, (1952). *Journal of Pediatrics*, **40**, 426–41

this is not essential. They are useful used repeatedly if the patient has a nutritional problem and can give some indication of when to expect the adolescent growth spurt which is heralded by a loss of limb fat and an equalling of the values for triceps and subscapular thicknesses.

The orchidometer (Fig. 2.6a) is held in one hand while the testes are palpated with the other. The standards for testicular volume are shown in Fig. 2.6b.

The tape measure is used to record occipito-frontal (head) circumference and can also be used to measure limb circumferences. The latter can be used to assess differential accumulation or loss of fat and muscle if combined with measurements of skinfold thickness.

Bone age

There are two widely used systems for estimating skeletal maturity, those of Greulich and Pyle (the atlas method) and of Tanner and Whitehouse (the rating method). Both are associated with appropriate prediction equations designed for use with *normal* children. The Tanner and Whitehouse calculations are tedious and, for pathological conditions, the fractions of growth achieved as described by Bayley and Pinneau (Table 2.1) are more robust; I use them in conjunction with Tanner and Whitehouse bone age scores tempered with a large degree of commonsense and caution (see below).

It does not matter which system of assessment of skeletal maturity is

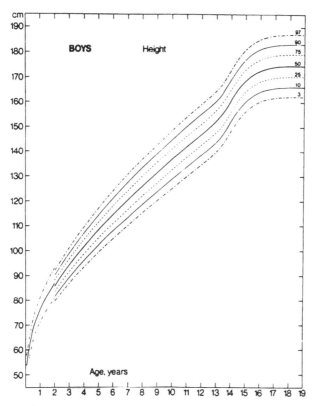

Fig. 2.7. Standard height centile chart.

used as long as the method is done properly and done repeatedly by the same observer. The proper method for each system is to examine each bone in the carpus in turn. Using the Greulich and Pyle method, the nearest radiographic picture is chosen from the Atlas and a bone age allotted; when all the relevant centres have been examined and aged, the ages are meaned to give an overall value.

In the Tanner and Whitehouse method, a score is allotted to each centre; the scores are summed and related to 50th centile values plotted against chronological age to give the bone age in exactly the same way as some clinicians speak of height age or weight age. These are not useful measurements, because there is no uniform adult height or weight with which to relate an earlier value, but bone age is a useful term because adult bones are uniformly fused; thus the nearer the bone age is to adult values, the more nearly is growth complete.

Charts

The standard distance height centile chart (Fig. 2.7) will be familiar to most clinicians. It is worth reiterating that the centiles mean what they say: 3 % of *normal* children have heights below or above the 3rd and 97th centile lines. The chart is simply a description of the heights of a standard population as it is with which the height of an individual can be compared.

Velocity centile charts are much more complicated because the implication of the centile values depends upon the measurement interval. Successive values have to have a mean, year after year, between + and − 0.8 standard deviations if a child is not to gain or lose ground with respect to its peers but the mathematical justification for this statement is not germane to this text. For child health and out-patient clinics, the Middlesex height velocity chart (Fig. 2.8) may be helpful.

The relevance of height velocity measurement to paediatric endocrine practice will emerge in the succeeding pages because it is the key to successful practice. It is worth emphasising here that the calculation of height velocity is only easy and a matter of routine if decimal ages are used for all purposes (see Table 2.2). This calculation may seem tedious, but it rapidly becomes ingrained, and there really is no alternative.

Charts (standards) are available for all anthropometric measurements. They are usually drawn as centiles or as standard deviations, depending on the distribution of the characteristic in question, but their use is uniform.

Growth assessment – the clinical consultation

Measurements are made routinely of:

- height
- sitting height
- weight
- triceps and subscapular skinfold thickness
- head circumference
- puberty ratings (see pages 60, 61)

On the first attendance, the heights of both parents should be *measured*. The value, if either of the heights is reported, is greatly reduced because of the tendency to report an idealized height of the spouse. (I have a theory that the heights of fathers are reported by mothers in relation to the esteem in which the child's father is held.)

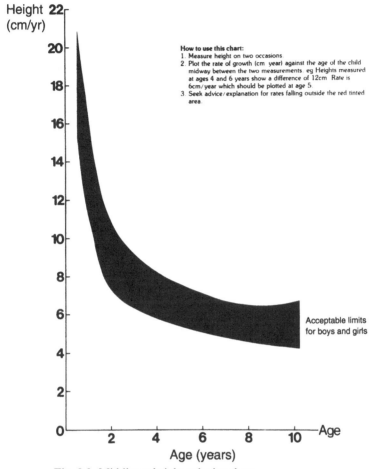

Fig. 2.8. Middlesex height velocity chart.

Birth data on the child and siblings should be gathered, together with measurement of the heights of siblings where possible. It is customary to ask about parental entry to puberty, usually as the age of maternal menarche; when the result accords with the physician's presumption, there is satisfaction all round but the contrary is not unusual, so the value of this question is doubtful except in a social context.

An assessment of skeletal maturity is likely to be helpful on this occasion.

The decimal age should be calculated, and the data either plotted on appropriate charts or calculated as standard deviation scores (Z-scores, SDS). The parental height centile positions should also be entered on the

Table 2.2. *Table of decimal dates*

To use this table, take today's date, 7th June 1993 (93.430) and subtract my birth date (15 January 1940, 40.038) to give my decimal age today (53.392).

	1 Jan.	2 Feb.	3 Mar.	4 Apr.	5 May	6 June	7 July	8 Aug.	9 Sept.	10 Oct.	11 Nov.	12 Dec.
1	000	085	162	247	329	414	496	581	666	748	833	915
2	003	088	164	249	332	416	499	584	668	751	836	918
3	005	090	167	252	334	419	501	586	671	753	838	921
4	008	093	170	255	337	422	504	589	674	756	841	923
5	011	096	173	258	340	425	507	592	677	759	844	926
6	014	099	175	260	342	427	510	595	679	762	847	929
7	016	101	178	263	345	430	512	597	682	764	849	932
8	019	104	181	266	348	433	515	600	685	767	852	934
9	022	107	184	268	351	436	518	603	688	770	855	937
10	025	110	186	271	353	438	521	605	690	773	858	940
11	027	112	189	274	356	441	523	608	693	775	860	942
12	030	115	192	277	359	444	526	611	696	778	863	945
13	033	118	195	279	362	447	529	614	699	781	866	948
14	036	121	197	282	364	449	532	616	701	784	868	951
15	038	123	200	285	367	452	534	619	704	786	871	953
16	041	126	203	288	370	455	537	622	707	789	874	956
17	044	129	205	290	373	458	540	625	710	792	877	959
18	047	132	208	293	375	460	542	627	712	795	879	962
19	049	134	211	296	378	463	545	630	715	797	882	964
20	052	137	214	299	381	466	548	633	718	800	885	967
21	055	140	216	301	384	468	551	636	721	803	888	970
22	058	142	219	304	386	471	553	638	723	805	890	973
23	060	145	222	307	389	474	556	641	726	808	893	975
24	063	148	225	310	392	477	559	644	729	811	896	978
25	066	151	227	312	395	479	562	647	731	814	899	981
26	068	153	230	315	397	482	564	649	734	816	901	984
27	071	156	233	318	400	485	567	652	737	819	904	986
28	074	159	236	321	403	488	570	655	740	822	907	989
29	077		238	323	405	490	573	658	742	825	910	992
30	079		241	326	408	493	575	660	745	827	912	995
31	082		244		411		578	663		830		997
	Jan. 1	Feb. 2	Mar. 3	Apr. 4	May 5	June 6	July 7	Aug. 8	Sept. 9	Oct. 10	Nov. 11	Dec. 12

growth chart to give an idea of whether or not the child is near to expected height for age for the family. If a boy's chart is being used, the mother's centile position will be plotted after adding 12.6 cm to her measured height. The father's height is entered directly. If a girl's chart is being used, the mother's height is entered directly but the height of the father must be adjusted by the subtraction of 12.6 cm to ascertain his centile position.

The skeletal maturity will give an index of how much growth has already occurred and thus how much is to come. Note that this is all the information it will give – the diagnostic yield is close to zero.

At a subsequent visit, the routine measurements will be repeated and it will be possible on this occasion to calculate the height velocity using the two decimal ages to calculate the time interval, and the two height measurements to calculate the gain. The result should either be plotted on a chart or the SDS calculated. Note that there is no point in relating height velocity to bone age – at least not unless there is a bone age increment and a height velocity related to the increment, and even then it has a suspect status. Why should they be related?

It is not possible to calculate height velocity SDS or plot the values over the age of 10 years in a girl or 11 years in a boy because of the effect of puberty on the standards. In the individual case, relating the velocity to the assessment of puberty is highly relevant.

With this knowledge it will be possible to sort out most disorders of growth in children.

The short child

All diseases impair growth so a child who is growing slowly needs a diagnosis and treatment. A child growing at a rate appropriate for his age and stature may need a diagnosis to explain why he is short but there is no point in seeking an active disease process through extensive investigation in such a patient. Whether treatment is possible or desirable is contentious and will be discussed below.

The clinical process

The starting point is growth assessment as already described. The height should be plotted on a distance centile chart both for chronological age and bone age. Parental centile positions should be entered after a correction has been applied to the measured height of the father or mother to make it appropriate for the sex of the child in question. Add 12.6 cm to the height of the mother to plot her height on a male centile chart: this will give the height she would have been had she been a man. The arithmetic mean of the parental heights adjusted for the sex of the child will give the target height centile and a range of ± 9 cm will include 95 % confidence limits of the expected adult height of the offspring. The reverse process applies to girls: subtract 12.6 cm from the measured height of the father etc.

Three possibilities now exist.

1. The child has the height one would expect for the children of these parents. One can predict the adult height and, assuming all goes well from now on, there is nothing more to say. The parents should be told what to expect in terms of growth in the next 6–12 months and asked to report back if things do not turn out as predicted.
2. The child is small for the parental centiles, but the bone age is delayed, so the predicted adult height is normal for the family. It is essential that the child be seen again on at least one occasion to make sure that the growth velocity is normal so that the predicted height will be achieved.
3. The child is small for the parental centiles and the predicted adult height is small for the family. This child needs a diagnosis. Treatment may be needed.

    CARE: This scheme of clinical management of the short child makes the assumption that the parents are normal. They may not be and the easiest mistake is wrongly to diagnose 'familial short stature'.

If either or both parents have heights less than the 3rd centile, measure their sitting heights (have they a skeletal dysplasia?). Take a history of stature in their first degree relatives (could they, as children, have had a growth problem which might have been remediable in the light of present knowledge and which might have been passed on to the child?).

Growth velocity

The measurement of growth velocity requires two measurements of stature made over a period of time which is long enough for more growth to have occurred than the cumulative error on the two measurements. If we assume that stature can be measured with an error of ± 2 mm, the cumulative error on two measurements is 8 mm. One should not, therefore, attempt to

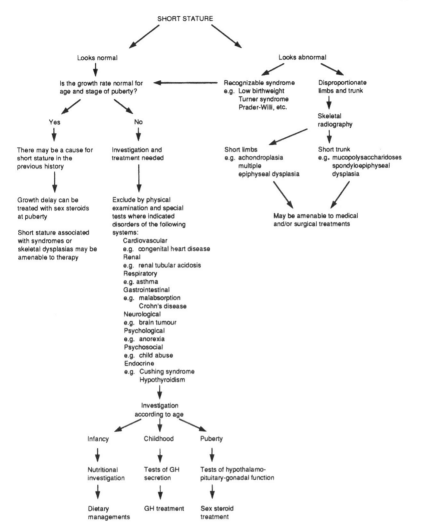

Fig. 2.9. Algorithm for the diagnosis of short stature.

record an increment in growth of much less than twice this figure or 1.6 cm. In the first year of life, a baby might achieve this in one month; in the teenage years it might take 4 months. A safe rule is not to place reliance on measurements made in childhood over less than 3 months, and to regard a velocity over such a short time with suspicion. If, for example, a child appeared to have grown 1.2 cm in 3 months, the velocity may be calculated as $1.2/0.25 = 4.8$ cm/year. However, with a maximal error of 8 mm, it could be as much as $2.0/0.25 = 8.0$ cm/year or as little as $0.4/0.25 =$

1.6 cm/year. The implications of these different figures could be very different in a child of any age.

In practice, a growth velocity calculated over a short period of time and related to the clinical situation may be obviously normal, obviously abnormal, or equivocal – and most likely to be the last and require repetition over a longer period of time. The longer a velocity remains below the 50th centile, the more likely it is that investigation will reveal an abnormality. If all children with growth velocities on or below the 25th centile over one year were to be investigated, 25% would yield normal results. The chance of a normal child growing for two successive years at this centile is around $0.25 \times 0.25 = 0.0625$, that is only 6.25% of children would be expected to yield normal results.

Even so, deciding what constitutes normality is the hardest task in clinical paediatric practice, let alone paediatric endocrinology. So much hangs upon the decision because it is possibly more reprehensible to investigate a normal child than not to investigate an abnormal one.

If in doubt, it is best to wait because the passage of time will usually reveal the true situation. The Middlesex height velocity chart shown in Fig. 2.8 can be used to give lower limits of what can be accepted for whole year velocities at different ages. Beyond the age of 10 years the slope of the lower line can be projected forwards but is only applicable to children who are showing no signs of development in puberty. The assessment of height velocity during puberty is important and difficult and will be covered in Chapter 3 (page 78).

Differential diagnosis

An algorithm for the management of a short child is shown in Fig. 2.9. Clinical examination should set the clinician off down the right track.

The child who looks normal

The key to how to proceed turns on the measurement of growth velocity which has been discussed. Growth velocity and its management in the context of late puberty will be covered in Chapter 3.

Normal growth velocity

It is doubtful whether anything can make a substantial difference to the final height of short children growing normally. There are trials of treatment with growth hormone running in such children at present; there is no doubt that growth hormone therapy will increase the height velocity of any child if sufficient doses are used, but this does not mean necessarily that the final height will be increased if the growing time is shortened. Growth hormone has a powerful influence on the gonads and increases the rate at which children go through puberty so the best estimates of efficacy in 1992 suggest that giving growth hormone to normal children may result in an increase in final stature of about 4 cm after 10 years of treatment, which hardly seems worthwhile. A possible way forward, which has not yet been tested, may be to use short, sharp courses of growth hormone for the short-term advantages which may accrue.

Growth hormone has also been used for the treatment of short stature associated with many other conditions, such as renal failure, skeletal dysplasias, Turner syndrome, Noonan syndrome, intrauterine growth retardation and others. Until the current carefully constituted trials of growth hormone in these conditions have reported final heights, there is no indication for the use of this treatment in the one-off situation.

Low growth velocity

By definition, an explanation must be found to explain a low growth velocity, and corrective treatment must be instituted as soon as possible because there will be cumulative loss of height potential if the skeletal maturity advances and the child does not grow adequately. The ideal situation, therefore, is to detect a poor growth velocity before it has a chance to cause short stature and to correct the abnormality.

Any paediatric disorder may present in this way so the clinician has to be alert to set off in the right investigative direction. Where he begins also depends upon the age of the patient he is investigating because of the different mechanisms controlling the growth process at different ages. In general, thinness is not usually a feature of endocrine diseases which affect growth, whereas it occurs frequently in the context of other causes of failure to thrive.

Under the age of one year, a low growth velocity is likely to be nutritional in origin and the remedy likely to be dietary in nature. It is important to realize that many problems associated with intrauterine growth retardation carry forward into feeding difficulties in the first year of life. The Silver–Russell syndrome is typical of this (and I do not accept the diagnosis without such a history) but, despite the feeding difficulty, the growth velocity is normal. At this time of life, perhaps beyond all others, the precept of 'first do no harm' is paramount.

I have seen many children investigated invasively and inappropriately,

Table 2.3. *Causes of growth hormone insufficiency*

Congenital	Acquired

Hereditary
  – due to gene deletion
Idiopathic GHRH deficiency
Developmental abnormalities
  – pituitary aplasia
  – pituitary hypoplasia
  – midline brain defects
	Tumours of hypothalamus or pituitary
	
	Other brain tumours
	Secondary to
	  – cranial irradiation
	  – head injury
	  – infection
	Transient due to
	  – low sex hormone concentration
	  – psychosocial deprivation

simply on the basis of being small or of having what is perceived to be a poor weight gain. It is my considered opinion that the world would not be a significantly worse place if weighing scales had never been invented; had they not been, children's lengths, which is what really matters, would be measured more frequently and more accurately than they are. Deciding whether a child has a nutritional status (weight) appropriate for his length can be done by eye or skinfold calipers. An infant should only be investigated if he is fail*ING* to thrive because only present and future growth velocity can be corrected; what is past is past.

In the childhood phase of growth, growth hormone secretion is the predominant influence on growth velocity. If clinical examination and appropriate investigation has excluded other diseases, it is appropriate to consider whether an insufficiency of growth hormone is causing a low growth velocity. The interpretation of the various tests of growth hormone secretion is difficult because most diseases impair growth hormone responsiveness to the usual stimuli (see Chapter 10, page 162). In Australasia, this has led to the abandonment of tests of growth hormone secretion as a prelude to the introduction of growth hormone treatment, which is perhaps going a little too far but it is a logical stance.

For the growth hormone insufficient child (Table 2.3), the use of growth hormone will restore a normal growth velocity after a period of catch-up growth (Fig. 2.10). GH insufficiency is the only definite indication for the use of GH at the time of writing. Because of the nature of the asymptotic relation between GH secretion and growth velocity, the smallest, most slowly growing and most severely GH-insufficient children will respond best and a reverse asymptote relates pretreatment GH secretory capacity

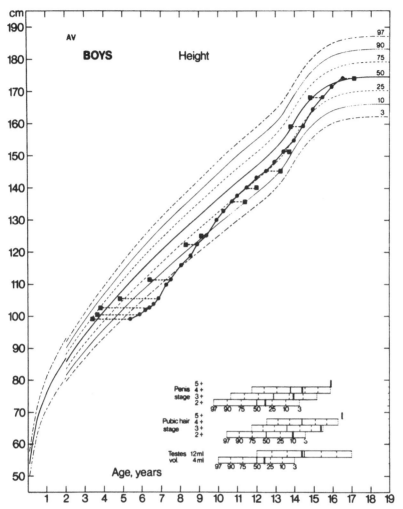

Fig. 2.10. Growth chart typical of GH insufficiency and the response to treatment.

and response to a given dose. Because of the nature of the original relationship, the response to GH treatment is inversely correlated to pretreatment height velocity so that it is possible to generate a series of dose–response curves relating pretreatment state, dose of GH and expected response (Fig. 2.11). A dose to achieve a desired acceleration appropriate for the individual can be selected from these curves, assuming that the skeleton is normal. Where it is not, for instance, due to Turner syndrome or a skeletal dysplasia, a bigger dose is required.

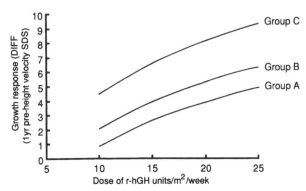

Fig. 2.11. Dose–response curves for GH treatment. Group C data are from children with clear evidence of GH insufficiency: a small dose of GH caused an impressive acceleration of height velocity. Group A was a group of short children growing normally for age and with normal GH secretion: they needed a much bigger dose to get a similar effect. Group B children had a pretreatment height velocity SDS between −0.8 and −2.0 and fulfilled the diagnostic criteria for 'partial' GH insufficiency. The importance of their curve is that it parallels the other two: the slopes are identical – only the intercepts differ. (From Darendeliler *et al.* (1990), *J. Endocr.* **125**, 311–16.)

If a child given GH fails to respond, much the most likely reasons are that he is not receiving the treatment, which is most likely, or that he has an occult skeletal dysplasia. A very few cases may have a true resistance to GH but they should have been identified before treatment by having a high basal serum GH concentration and a low IGF-1 concentration (Fig. 2.12). Antibodies to exogenously administered GH are a thing of the past, except in those very rare cases of true GH *DE*ficiency due to deletion of the GH gene as opposed to GH insufficiency, which is usually the result of pituitary hypoplasia secondary to GHRH *INSUF*ficiency.

For children of pubertal age but without signs of puberty, a low growth velocity nearly always indicates a prolongation of growth at a childhood rate along the childhood curve without the take-off of the pubertal curve. The remedy for this is administration of sex steroids (see Chapter 3, page 82). The interpretation of GH responsiveness to the usual stimuli in such a patient is notoriously difficult. If the temptation to perform a test cannot be resisted, the child should be given a priming dose of sex steroids two days before the test (testosterone 100 mg or ethinyl estradiol 30 μg).

In a child who is showing secondary sex characteristics appropriate for an increase in growth rate (Breast stage 2, testicular volumes > 8 ml) which is not occurring, it is possible that he or she has an inability to increase the

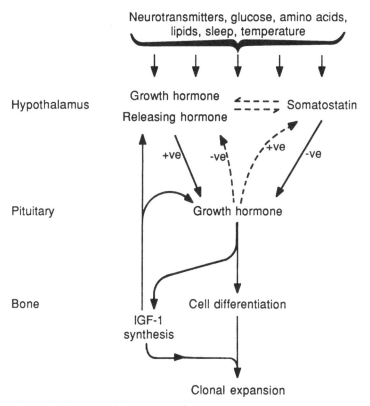

Neurotransmitters, glucose, amino acids,
lipids, sleep, temperature

Hypothalamus — Growth hormone Releasing hormone ← – – – → Somatostatin

+ve -ve +ve -ve

Pituitary — Growth hormone

Bone — IGF-1 synthesis   Cell differentiation

Clonal expansion

Fig. 2.12. The growth hormone axis.

amplitude of pulsatile GH secretion for any of the reasons shown in Table 2.3. In such patients it is appropriate to investigate the GH reserve with an unprimed test and to administer GH if indicated.

The child who does not look normal

The diagnosis of recognizable patterns of malformation (dysmorphology) reaches its apogee in computer-assisted data banks. The clinician should not be daunted by this sort of jargon beloved of Departments of Genetics. There are some syndromes, such as Silver–Russell, Turner, Prader–Willi, Noonan, etc, which occur sufficiently commonly to be required knowledge but the more abstruse syndromes require access to an appropriate text or computer programme. In terms of the management of the symptoms of these diagnoses, and especially of the growth disorders which are so frequently associated, the steps to take are *exactly* the same as they are for any other child, the assessment of growth velocity and the application of the appropriate remedy for age. These children do not need to be made exceptions to the normal rules for treatment.

The *Turner syndrome* needs a special mention. All patients who are diagnosed after birth have lost the paternal second sex chromosome: loss of the maternal X chromosome is a lethal deletion. The phenotype of patients with Turner syndrome is remarkably uniform regardless of the genotype: the reason is probably that a complete deletion of the second sex chromosome in every cell line is lethal so that all patients have mosaic karyotypes, even if the karyotype in the blood lymphocytes is 45X. Of patients seen with the Turner syndrome, approximately 50 % have a 45X karyotype in the blood and the remainder have combinations of ring, isochromosomes and mixed patterns in a variety of combinations. If one studies more than one tissue, the incidence of mosaicism rises to 70 % in the case of two tissues, 90 % in the case of three tissues and so on. This is probably why the phenotype is so similar.

Patients are born small for dates. They may be detectable at birth because of lymphedema: the abnormality of lymphatic drainage is very conspicuous in the fetal period (and may recur with estrogen at puberty) and the compression caused by the accumulation of lymph is widely held to be responsible for many if not all of the congenital abnormalities which are common, such as neck webbing, coarctation, renal abnormalities (often leading to hypertension later) and the conspicuous nail changes (Fig. 2.13), which often give a clue to the diagnosis in later childhood.

Turner girls have specific feeding difficulties in the infantile period and lose more growth during the first year of life. They grow consistently at a 25th centile velocity during childhood, which leads to a further gradual loss of stature. The patients have a severe mesenchymal defect which is manifest in the skeletal dysplasia characteristic of the syndrome: the long bones show a coarse trabecular pattern and the vertebrae are relatively tall for the stature. Like all patients with skeletal dysplasia, patients with the Turner syndrome grow very badly in the pubertal years whether they have a natural puberty or have it induced artificially.

The consequence of these several growth deficits is a cumulative loss of about 20 cm from the height one might predict from the heights of the parents. The correlation between the height of a girl with Turner syndrome and her parental heights is identical to normal: there is simply a loss of a constant amount of height. Thus the Turner offspring of tall parents will attain a short normal final height.

There is much debate about the treatment of the short stature of Turner

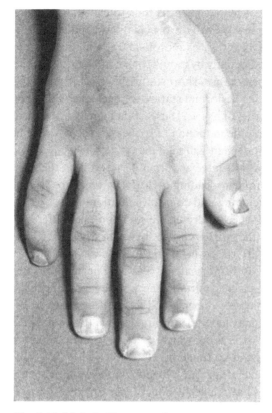

Fig. 2.13. Nails in Turner syndrome.

syndrome and no final conclusions in 1993. Sex steroids, anabolic steroids and growth hormone have all been used over the years to increase height velocity of Turner patients during the childhood phase of growth. They are all effective in achieving this aim. GH has a marginal advantage because, used in high doses (30 + units/m²/week in daily divided doses), it does not, as do the steroids, cause excessive skeletal maturation. For this reason GH has become accepted as the major therapeutic tool; for those who do not have access to it, it should be remembered that it is not the only tool and that the longest running series are reporting final heights only around the bottom of the normal female adult range of height. This is obviously an improvement on the final predicted Turner height but it is not normal and it is not as high as some clinicians have predicted because, no matter how they are managed, patients with the Turner syndrome do not grow normally during the pubertal years.

A practical course of management is thus to encourage feeding in the infantile period, to follow growth during childhood and to introduce GH, low dose anabolic steroids (e.g. oxandrolone 0.625 mg daily) or low dose estrogen (1–2 µg estradiol daily by mouth) or a combination of the first two when the growth velocity causes short stature which is disadvantageous to the child. If she remains of normal stature for age, given that GH is most effective in the early years of its use, I suspect that it may be best to add GH just before, and during the induction of, puberty to achieve the best final result. Proof of this statement will take many years more.

The management of associated abnormalities is without the scope of this text but middle ear problems leading to deafness, renal abnormalities and hypertension need excluding and constant attention.

Patients with the Turner syndrome have a number of different gonadal problems: in infancy the gonads can be streak, in which case the LH and FSH concentrations are raised in the newborn period and this is worth documenting. They may be normal and may stay normal for some years: 20% of girls with Turner syndrome show some spontaneous onset of puberty, although complete puberty and fertility are much less frequent than this. The ovaries may have an appearance on ultrasound intermediate between normal and streak, in which case the gonadotrophin concentrations are the best guide to function.

During the 12th year of life, all patients with elevated gonadotrophin concentrations should have puberty induced (see Chapter 10, page 171). If the LH and FSH concentrations are low, it is permissible to wait a while for spontaneous ovarian activity and this should be sought with pelvic ultrasonography. Induction of puberty should not be much later than the 12th birthday under any circumstances. This is because a slow induction with estrogens, and adequate and concomitant endogenous or exogenous GH, is required to grow the normal uterus which may be required for later embryo transfer. If there is a Y chromosomal cell line, the dysgenetic gonads should be removed during the teenage years if not before.

The question of infertility should be raised with the parents and, probably through them with the child if they are willing, very early in childhood. Adult infertile women recommend that the first time the child talks about her own babies, she should be told (at her own level) that conceiving will be a problem so that she grows up accustomed to the unpleasant reality of the position. The message must not land on an unsuspecting teenager and teenagers must not be expected to interpret accurately statements about 'inactive ovaries'; adolescents do not associate the acquisition of secondary sexual characteristics with reproductive capability (which may be why initial sexual adventures are so often unplanned and, more importantly in these days of AIDS, unprotected).

Disproportionate short stature

The measurement of standing and sitting heights may reveal the cause of short stature but diagnosis depends critically upon the interpretation of skeletal radiographs which depends, in turn, upon close collaboration with an interested radiologist, of which there are few and even fewer with experience. Reported radiographic diagnoses by non-experts should be regarded with suspicion.

Treatments for skeletal dysplasias with short trunks are very unrewarding; the position with regard to medical treatments (GH) for short limbs is currently *sub judice* but one is sometimes pleasantly surprised by a growth response to GH in a patient with achondroplasia, especially in the youngest patients. Long term results are not yet available. Surgical limb lengthening shows increasing promise for patients with short limbs but is, for them, a formidable undertaking in terms of time and discomfort. I think that such procedures should not be undertaken until the child itself is able itself to express an opinion.

The tall child

The algorithm for the elucidation of the problem of tall stature is shown in Fig. 2.14. The therapeutic emphasis in this situation is usually directed at subverting a normal process (limiting adult stature) which is a somewhat unusual position for the physician to adopt. An exception to such a rule is found in the management of precocious puberty which will be addressed in Chapter 3.

Tall children become tall and become tall adults by growing continuously at a rate greater than their smaller peers. The assessment of what constitutes normality is thus similar to the assessment of an abnormal velocity in a small child, which has been discussed. Pointers to seek an explanation include a growth rate year on year greater than the 90th centile, a height attained which is greater than one might expect for the family and a height prediction which is increasing inexorably.

The methods of height prediction have been considered previously: the most robust has been shown repeatedly to be that of Bayley and Pinneau. In view of the difficulties and potential dangers of limiting adult stature, I am reluctant even to discuss treatment with a height prediction of less than

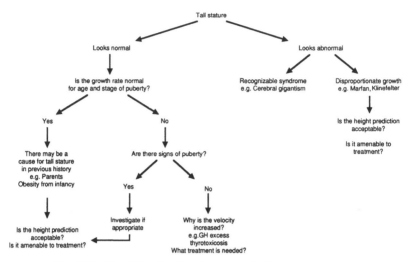

Fig. 2.14. Algorithm for the diagnosis of tall stature.

200 cm for a boy or 180 cm for a girl – and these limits are rising year by year.

For an adult, however, tall stature seems to be more of a handicap than short stature. Small parents will bring their small, normal children for a consultation and be quite surprised to see how short they are themselves in relation to the adult population. It is often the children themselves, the school or people outside the family who initiate the consultation. Tall children , on the other hand, have a considerable advantage at school and in sport and often find it difficult to understand why they are dragged to a doctor for a problem which they do not perceive.

Tall parents will then regale the physician with appalling stories of the misery caused by their excessive stature, especially during the teenage years. They also complain of the embarrassment of (for them) short beds, low doors, badly designed modes of transport, difficulty in buying shoes and clothes and, worst of all, the remarks that are addressed to them by strangers in the street.

I conclude that short stature is disadvantageous to children but a state with which it is possible to become accustomed in adult life. Tall stature is advantageous to the child but a serious handicap in terms of social life to an adult: the problem for such a person cannot be ignored.

(a)

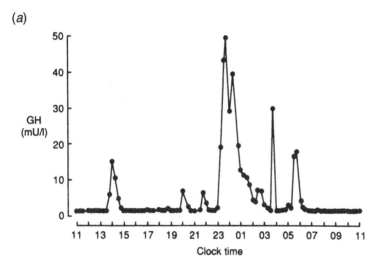

(b)

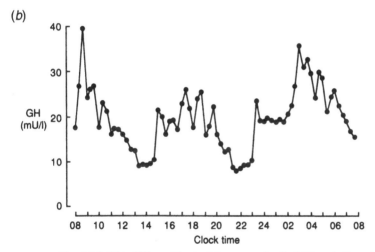

Fig. 2.15. 24 h GH profiles in (a) a normal tall child and (b) a child with gigantism. Note the failure of the GH to return to baseline in (b). Although the growth velocity of the children was similar, the output of growth hormone is greatly increased in (b), demonstrating an inefficient use of non-pulsatile GH.

Differential diagnosis

When precocious puberty, thyrotoxicosis and an exaggerated response to adrenal androgens have been excluded in a normal looking child, the chief question is to define gigantism and to differentiate it from the hormonal pattern of GH secretion seen in a normal tall child. In the case of profiles such as those shown in Fig. 2.15, the failure of the GH level ever to return to the baseline is unmistakable – and the child proved to have a GH secreting adenoma of the pituitary which was successfully and selectively removed by transphenoidal surgery.

It is not always so obvious and so the tests of normal GH control used in the diagnosis and management of acromegaly in older patients (failure of suppression of GH after glucose load, a paradoxical response to administration of thyrotrophin releasing hormone or gonadotrophin releasing hormone, etc.) have been tried in paediatrics. Unfortunately, the performance of such tests is more difficult in the context of the increased activity of the pituitary in the normal child, let alone the tall one. If glucose were to be administered just after a spontaneous burst of GH secretion had occurred, the concentration would fall regardless of the stimulus because there would be no GH readily releasable from the pituitary. The failure of the GH level to fall may, therefore, be a useful indicator of abnormal GH control but a 'normal' result does not ensure normality. The analysis of the GH profile, a raised IGF-1 concentration and, most importantly, the clinical situation, should be the pointers to imaging procedures (Fig. 2.16).

Our experience of selective petrosal sinus sampling for GH with and without the administration of GHRH has been rather disappointing in terms of lateralizing a putative GH adenoma by hormonal tests. We have had the same disappointing experience with CRH and ACTH in the localization of a basophil adenoma in childhood Cushing disease. I assume that this must be attributed to the increased vascularity and mixing of blood from both sides in children as opposed to adults.

Klinefelter syndrome and other syndromes involving additional sex chromosomal material need a special mention in terms of diagnosis. These children gain a constant amount of height in relation to the heights of the family (just as 45X children lose it) but a special problem occurs in those with excessive X chromosomal material whose testes produce inadequate amounts of testosterone at puberty because such patients, who may not necessarily have grown excessively in childhood, simply go on growing, seemingly indefinitely. They become increasingly easier to identify and diagnose with a karyotype examination but it is then too late to lose height already gained.

The hallmark of these children is their body proportions in earlier childhood (they have excessively long legs even before puberty), the small size of the penis and the unusually soft texture of the testes on palpation. Gynecomastia is the well-known sign of inadequate testosterone production at puberty but the condition should have been recognized before

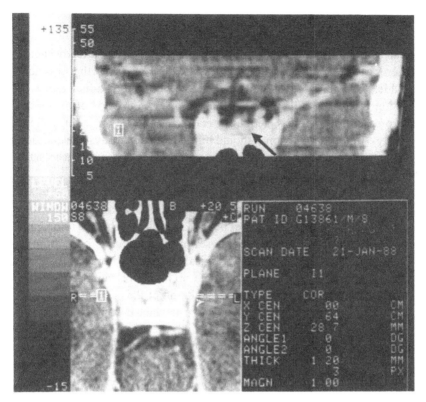

Fig. 2.16. CT appearance of GH secreting adenoma.

this occurs because, once it has done so (and it is preventable with early introduction of testosterone), it requires surgical correction by subareolar mastectomy, sometimes even plastic surgery. A karyotype examination should be an early test in the investigation of any child unusually tall for the family, especially if he manifests learning difficulties.

Marfan syndrome has characteristic cardiovascular and ocular manifestations as well as long-limbed, tall stature with arachnodactyly. It appears to be caused by mutations in a single fibrillin gene on chromosome 15 which could be important both for diagnosis and for antenatal prevention. The cardiac abnormalities are not related to this chromosome (or to the fibrillin gene on chromosome 5) but are a major cause of death. All children with Marfan syndrome should have regular echocardiography of the mitral valve and aortic root at annual intervals from their teenage years.

Treatment

In tall stature, prevention is better than cure; losing height already gained requires complex and hazardous surgery so, the earlier growth assessment is made, the better are the long term prospects of limiting adult stature. A decision to treat a tall child will be made first on grounds of diagnosis. Thyrotoxicosis obviously requires treatment and so does precocious puberty. A pituitary adenoma should be removed surgically. The question is what to do for the other (much more numerous) children who have excessive predicted adult heights.

The mainstay of traditional treatment has been the introduction of sex steroids before they would otherwise be expected to arise by endogenous secretion, i.e. the early induction of puberty. This has been done using large doses of estrogens in girls or large doses of testosterone in boys, both of which treatments employ unphysiological doses which may carry long-term side effects. Such treatments should no longer be employed.

Since their rationale is to induce the take-off of the puberty component of growth at a point on the childhood curve at which it would not normally be expected to occur in the individual child, there can be no need to use doses of sex steroids greater than would normally be employed for the induction of puberty. It will be necessary to get to adult replacement doses more quickly than one would do in a small child; one takes it slowly in such a patient to allow time for growth to occur during the induction of puberty, which is exactly what one wishes to avoid in the tall child for the limitation of growth.

The scheme shown on page 171 should therefore be introduced when the child is 30 cm away from the desired final height and the final doses should be reached by a rapid increase taking not less than six months to achieve them. Theoretically, one should be able to avoid the major side effects of sex steroid administration, although the long-term consequences of taking estrogen by mouth have not been adequately assessed in any groups of patients, least of all these.

Because of the anxiety about the long-term effects of early exposure to sex steroids, especially to estrogens, and most especially to the large doses which have been conventional, my colleagues and I have been trying alternative strategies based on the idea of limiting growth velocity during the childhood phase of growth by reducing endogenous GH scretion. Our early attempts at using the anticholinergic agents, such as atropine or pirenzepine, were successful in their primary aim but the side effects were unpleasant. We also became concerned at the theoretical effect of such agents on short term memory, which might impair school performance. Most importantly, the reduction in growth velocity seemed to require increasing doses and the effect on height prediction was trivial. This was probably because we used them during the years of puberty when a reduction of predicted height has been especially difficult to achieve by any means. We have therefore begun to investigate the use of an alternative agent, somatostatin, of which a long acting analogue (Octreotide®, Sandoz) is available.

Theoretically, this could be used in two ways, first to reduce the quantity of growth achieved during the childhood phase of growth and, secondly, to limit GH secretion and thereby the growth spurt achieved during puberty, allowing the endogenous sex steroids to do the job of hastening epiphyseal closure and thereby limiting the final stature attained. Of the fact that the treatment works, we are now in no doubt, assuming the side effects can be tolerated by the individual (abdominal pain and diarrhoea), which has not always been the case. It is too early to judge long term efficacy and therefore this modality of treatment cannot yet be safely recommended but it is in prospect.

Surgical treatments have been employed in the past but I do not recommend them. The stapling of epiphyses in particular seems to be quite ineffective and operations to reduce bone length should be very rarely employed.

The fat child

Obesity is so common in our society that a physician can make it more or less a part of his clinical practice as he chooses. There is no absolute threshold where fatness becomes pathological so what constitutes obesity varies according to the observer. Actuarial risk is not a bad starting place since obese adults have increased risks of death from cardiovascular disease, largely secondary to hypertension, and from diabetes mellitus. The persistence of obesity from childhood to adult life is notorious so this is a symptom which may be presented in the guise of an endocrine problem. It rarely turns out so to be and, whatever the cause, the remedy is far from straightforward.

The causes of obesity are shown in Table 2.4. The ones associated with endocrine pathology are generally characterized by short stature, or a low growth velocity in the initial stages, and sometimes by mental retardation as well. In endocrine terms the management starts with growth assessment. Measurements of height, height velocity and skinfold thickness are helpful,

Table 2.4. *Causes of obesity*

Aetiology	Examples	Comment
Dysmorphic or genetic	Prader–Willi Laurence–Moon–Biedl Down syndrome	Characterized by shortness and mental retardation
Endocrine	Hypothalamic Hypopituitary Hypogonad Cushing syndrome Hypothyroidism Pseudohypoparathyroidism Hyperinsulinemia	Characterized by shortness or puberty problems May have fits Hypoglycemia
Nutritional	'Simple' obesity	Characterized by tallness if of origin in infancy
Iatrogenic	Glucocorticoids Estrogens	
Inactivity Socio-economic	Spina bifida Low social class Ethnic	

particularly if they are made longitudinally. Weight measurements are unhelpful: one does not need any tools other than eyes to diagnose obesity and, in terms of follow-up, growth in height may make a weight standstill entirely appropriate to the therapeutic end.

The most intractable problems are those where hypothalamic function is disorganized, particularly after intracranial surgery. These patients and those with a congenital hypothalamic problem, such as the Prader–Willi syndrome, deserve especial sympathy – and sympathy is truthfully about all the physician has to offer. The Prader–Willi syndrome is diagnosed by history (floppiness and feeding difficulties in the newborn period) and clinical examination (typical facies, hands and feet). The diagnosis is confirmed by demonstrating deletion of genetic material from the long arm of the (paternally derived) chromosome 15.

Management

Starving people lose weight and a patient who does not lose weight on a particular diet has to eat less, which is easier said than done.

The quintessence of the dietary problem is revealed in some very simple mathematics. If I wish to lose 3 kg of adipose tissue, I need to generate a calorie deficit of $3000 \times 9 = 27000$ kcal. If I can stand the difficulty and boredom of eating a 1200 kcal diet, I might possibly contribute 6–800 kcal/24 h towards this total. In other words, at that rate (which I personally should find near impossible to maintain), it would take me between 33 and 45 days, 5 to 6 weeks, to generate a sufficient calorie deficit to achieve the loss of adipose tissue required, not to mention the complexity of the contribution of the loss of lean body mass to measured weight loss. Longitudinal skinfold measurements are likely to give a much better guide to progress than measurements of weight.

For a child who has an endocrine problem, and who is commenced on replacement therapy, the combination of increased energy requirements through better well-being and restored growth and development, as well as increased basal metabolic rate may assist the loss of adipose tissue if the patient continues to eat the same amount as before. All this can easily be negated if the calorie intake is increased.

For the same reason, a patient who starts a replacement or therapeutic regimen involving steroid hormones, particularly glucocorticoids or estrogens, both of which stimulate appetite, should be warned of the dangers of weight gain if care is not taken.

Increased physical activity is sometimes regarded as an attractive alternative to calorie restriction in the energy balance equation but it is a two-edged weapon. On the one hand, the laws of thermodynamics certainly act in the patient's favour but, on the other, increased exercise also stimulates appetite and the result may, therefore, not be so favourable. Also, without considerable energy expenditure (many miles of running a day), the contribution of exercise is limited at best.

The thin child

Unintentional loss of weight is rightly recognized as a serious problem but, as Table 2.5 indicates, it is seldom if ever associated with primary endocrine disease. On the other hand, the consequences to growth and development of unrecognized systemic or of psychological disease or socio-economic deprivation are considerable. These problems may present to the physician in the guise of an endocrine problem (short stature or delayed puberty) and the identification of the cause without resorting to elaborate tests is sometimes a real challenge to clinical skill. The discipline of growth assessment and what to do about the results will avoid many pitfalls.

Table 2.5. *Causes of thinness*

Aetiology	Examples	Characteristics
Syndromes	Lipodystrophy	
	Marfan	Tall
	Low birthweight	Body asymmetry
Organic disease	Paediatric problems	Short stature
Psychological	Anorexia nervosa	Short stature and/or
	Bulimia	delayed puberty
	Emotional deprivation	
Socio-economic	Inadequate or inedible	
	calories provided	

Management

Longitudinal measurements of height and skinfold thickness are invaluable, since the child who is thin but not getting thinner and who is growing at a normal rate does not need a diagnosis. To seek one is meddlesome, expensive and constitutes bad medical practice. The reverse is also true and, once a diagnosis has been established, treatment should be monitored with the same tools.

Once again, measurements of weight serve badly and particularly badly in the context of anorexia nervosa; in this condition, weight targets may be regarded by the patient as absolute rather than relative so that, as soon as she starts to grow or to develop in puberty she may exceed her target weight and yet be just as ill as ever. A skinfold thickness target is much more helpful to the growing child.

In the context of exercise- or calorie-induced gonadotrophin insufficiency and pubertal delay, the question is sometimes asked whether the administration of sex steroids for the induction of puberty can be helpful. This is a very difficult situation with which to deal because sex steroids have many beneficial effects on the physical side but many potentially deleterious effects on the emotional side. I always take second place to professional psychiatric advice in deciding the course to follow.

3
Puberty

Normal puberty and its endocrine control

The hypothalamo-pituitary-gonadal axis (Fig. 3.1) is functional in the fetus, and the effects of its lack can be seen in inadequate male development. Shortly after birth, concentrations of sex steroids and gonadotrophins are in the adult range, and they gradually reduce over the early months of life. They are easily stimulable at this age.

It seems clear that there is both positive and negative feedback in the system so that maternal hormones prime the axis and their withdrawal at birth spurs it into endogenous activity. During the childhood years, pulsatile GnRH secretion reduces, but the system is not as inactive as it was once thought to be. Measurement of 24 h hormonal profiles reveals that young children have occasional bursts of nocturnal gonadotrophin secretion, which increase in frequency and amplitude as the years go by, long before the signs of secondary sexual characteristics appear (Fig. 3.2). It is presumed that these changes arise secondarily to maturation of the GnRH pulse generator.

Activity can also be observed in ovarian morphology and in uterine size seen in ultrasonographic pelvic examination of girls during the childhood and pubertal years (Fig. 3.3). The prepubertal ovary is a small ovoid structure with a few small follicles; as soon as nocturnal pulsatile gonadotrophin secretion becomes established, the morphology becomes multicystic. 24 h gonadotrophin secretion allows the development of a dominant follicle which will ovulate when an LH surge is generated.

The uterus (Fig. 3.4) responds to the resulting estradiol secretion by changing from a tubular structure, in which the widest diameter is seen at the cervix, to a pear shaped structure with the body now having dimensions greater than the cervix. The endometrial echo becomes increasingly evident

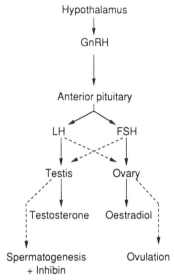

Fig. 3.1. Hypothalamo-pituitary–gonadal axis.

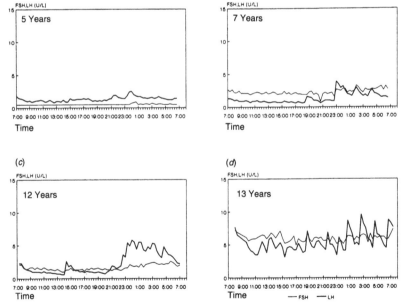

Fig. 3.2. 24 h gonadotrophin profiles (LH and FSH) in (*a*) prepuberty, (*b*) late prepuberty, (*c*) early puberty (*d*) late puberty. Note the progression of occasional pulsatile gonadotrophin secretion to nocturnal secretion to 24 h secretion.

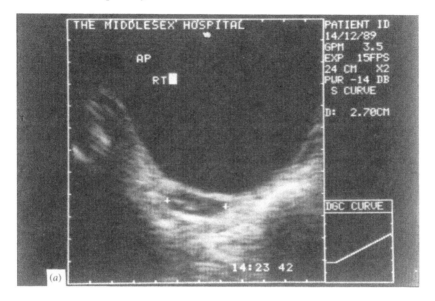

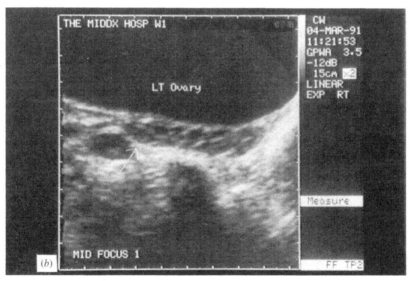

Fig. 3.3. Pelvic ultrasound image of (*a*) prepubertal ovary and (*b*) pubertal ovary showing multicystic change.

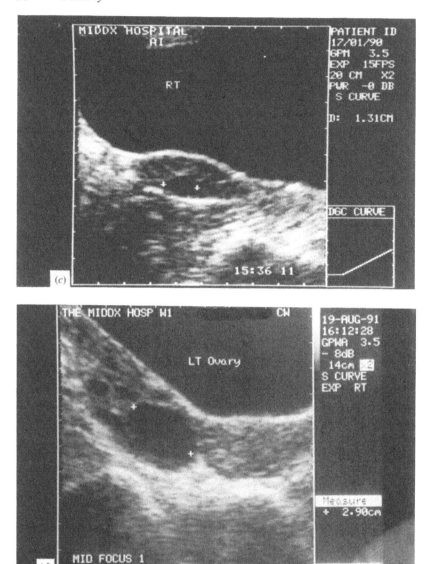

Fig. 3.3. Pelvic ultrasound image of (c) mature ovary showing a lead (dominant) follicle and (d) mature ovary showing a dominant follicle.

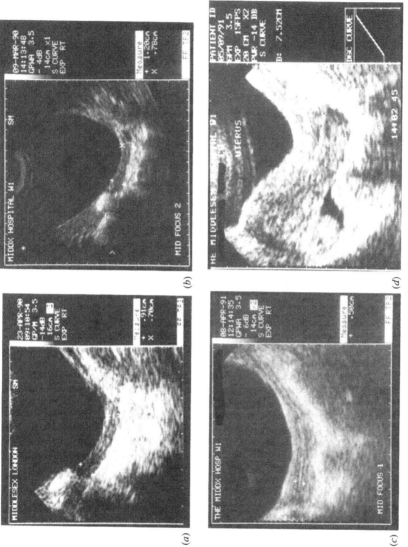

Fig. 3.4. Pelvic ultrasound images of the uterus (a) prepubertal (b) in early puberty, (c) in later puberty, premenarcheal, (d) adult pattern.

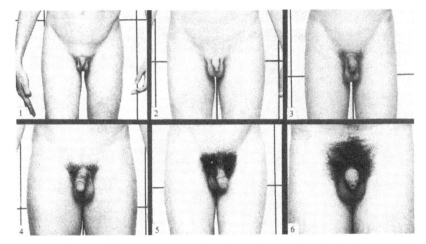

Fig. 3.5. Tanner stages of puberty for males. Genitalia stage 1: Preadolescent: testes, scrotum and penis are of about the same size and proportion as in early childhood. 2: Enlargement of scrotum and testes. Skin of scrotum reddens and changes in texture. Little or no enlargement of penis at this stage. 3: Enlargement of penis, which occurs at first mainly in length. Further growth of testes and scrotum. 4: Increased size of penis with growth in breadth and development of glans. Testes and scrotum larger; scrotal skin darkened. 5: Genitalia adult size and shape. Pubic hair stage 1: Preadolescent. The vellus over the pubes is not further developed than that over the abdominal wall, i.e. no pubic hair. 2: Sparse growth of long, slightly pigmented downy hair, straight or slightly curly, chiefly at the base of the penis. 3: Considerably darker, coarser and more curled. The hair spreads sparsely over the junction of the pubes. 4: Hair now adult in type, but area covered is still considerably smaller than in the adult. No spread to the medial surface of the thighs. 5: Adult in quantity and type with distribution of the horizontal (or classically 'feminine') pattern. Spread to medial surface of thighs. 6: Spread of pubic hair up linea alba.

as girls mature but menarche is unusual before a 5 mm endometrial thickness.

Secondary sexual characteristics

The Tanner stages of puberty for boys and girls are shown in Figs. 3.5 and 3.6, and the ages and ranges at which they appear are shown in Fig. 3.7. The measurement of testicular volume is accomplished using an orchidometer, and this instrument and the standards applicable to its use were shown in Fig. 2.6 (pp. 26, 27).

The first outward sign of puberty in a girl is the appearance of the breast bud. As soon as there is sufficient estradiol circulating to be manifest as

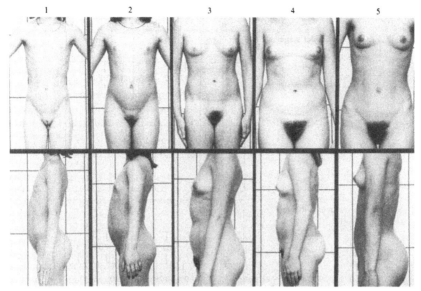

Fig. 3.6. Tanner stages of puberty for females. Breast stage 1: Preadolescent: elevation of papilla only. 2: Breast bud stage: elevation of breast and papilla as small mound. Enlargement of areola diameter. 3: Further enlargement and elevation of breast and areola with no separation of their contours. 4: Projection of areola and papilla to form a secondary mound above the level of the breast. 5: Mature stage: projection of papilla only, due to recession of the areola to the general contour of the breast. Pubic hair stages 1–5 as for males.

this, the growth rate starts to increase rapidly because of an increase in the amplitude of pulsatile GH secretion. The growth rate reaches a maximum of about 8 cm/year during breast stages 2 and 3, and then begins to decline as breast stage 4 is attained. As it does so, and at this breast (and pubic hair) stage, menarche occurs at a growth velocity of about 4 cm/year.

Pubic and axillary hair growth in girls is a manifestation of adrenal androgen secretion; it is not infrequent to see a scanty growth of hair and for a complaint to be made of apocrine sweat in children of either sex between the ages of 7 and 9. This has been called premature adrenarche (or sometimes premature pubarche) but the adjective applied is quite inappropriate since adrenarche is a physiological event in mid-childhood. It is obviously important to consider whether such a patient has an abnormal source of androgens (see Chapter 5) but the measurement of blood pressure to exclude Cushing syndrome and the relative paucity of signs of virilization (especially clitoromegaly and serious acne) is comforting.

During puberty, breast and pubic hair development usually proceed

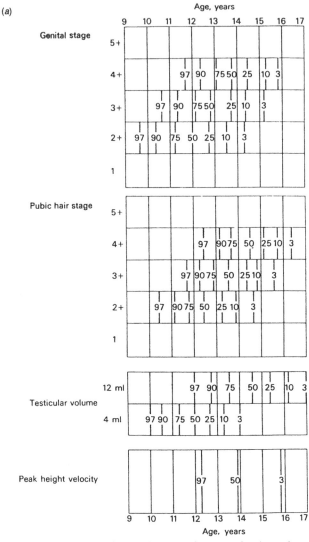

Fig. 3.7. (*a*). Centiles for attainment of stages of puberty in males.

roughly in parallel. I presume that estradiol has some facilitative action on hair follicle response to androgen secretion because a scanty growth of pubic hair is common in a girl with Turner syndrome who has received no treatment: as soon as a small dose of estradiol is introduced, pubic hair grows rapidly. It is unusual to see menarche before pubic hair stage 4.

The first sign of puberty in a boy is the change in the appearance of the penis and the enlargement of the testes. It is generally held that a testicular

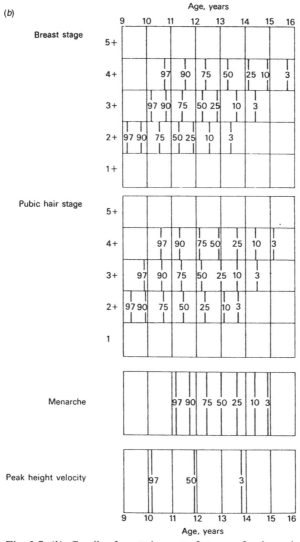

Fig. 3.7. (*b*). Centiles for attainment of stages of puberty in females.

volume of 4 ml is the outward manifestation of nocturnal pulsatile gonadotrophin secretion in a boy and this may well be correct. On the other hand, there is no doubt that the genitalia of boys begin to change before this age, and the prepubertal 2 ml testis can be perceived to attain a 3 ml volume with some change in penile appearance before true puberty becomes established. Indeed, I regard it as somewhat concerning if this does not happen.

While genitalia and pubic hair stages advance in parallel as testicular volume enlarges and testosterone levels rise, growth continues along the (decelerating) childhood curve. The contribution of adrenal androgens is trivial compared to the noise coming from the testes. The shape of the childhood curve dictates that a boy of 14 years with early puberty will not grow at a rate much more than 4 cm/year, and this decreases as age advances so that the growth of a boy of 16 in early puberty may be nearly stationary. Such patients show very little growth hormone response to any stimulus, and testing the growth hormone axis is liable to lead to an inappropriate diagnosis of GH insufficiency by the unwary. If it is felt essential to perform such a test, the patient will need to be primed by administration of testosterone before the test procedure (see Chapter 10). Growth hormone is the last therapy a patient with 'simple' delay of puberty requires. GH promotes local IGF-1 production which augments FSH action and increases LH receptors. Thus it accelerates puberty and epiphyseal closure (in both sexes) and may thereby compromise final height.

The delay in take-off of the pubertal spurt in a boy is attributed to two factors. The first is that testosterone is a much less effective stimulator of GH responsiveness than estradiol and presumably has to be aromatized in the hypothalamus to have its stimulatory effect on this axis. The second is that estradiol is anabolic at a relatively lower concentration than testosterone, even though the effect of testosterone at the level it achieves around stage 4 of genital and pubic hair development, and at a testicular volume of 10 ml, is obviously greater than that of estradiol.

As Fig. 2.4 showed, the peak of the adolescent growth spurt is greater and later in a boy than in a girl and this gains him about 5 cm in final height. Boys gain a further 10 cm by growing at a prepubertal rate along the childhood curve before the take-off of the puberty component but they lose about 2.4 cm through stopping growing more quickly than girls after the peak of their adolescent growth spurt. Although the take-off of pubertal growth is 2 years later in a boy than a girl, the cessation of growth is only one year later, so the 12.6 cm difference in the adult heights of men and women comprises 10 cm of growth at a prepubertal rate plus 5 cm of peak height velocity minus 2.4 cm of post peak growth (Fig. 3.8).

The facts that breast development is more obvious to the casual observer than penile enlargement and that a 12 year-old girl is taller than a 12 year old boy are, I believe, the reason why girls are generally considered to mature earlier than boys: Fig. 3.7 shows that the difference in timing of the onset of puberty is actually trivial. It is true that testes probably require a

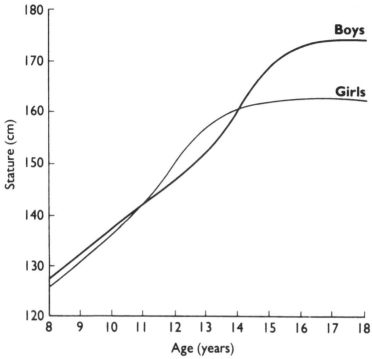

Fig. 3.8. Heights attained during the adolescent growth spurt in boys and girls.

higher level of gonadotrophin stimulation than ovaries, which is why early puberty is commoner in girls, and late puberty commoner in boys, but the perceived wisdom that girls enter puberty ahead of boys is not correct. Nor do girls attain reproductive capability earlier than boys: spermarche (finding sperm in early morning specimens of urine) occurs at about the same age as menarche but most perimenarcheal cycles are anovulatory and remain irregular for about 18 months, so boys are generally technically capable of fathering a child before girls are capable of conceiving one.

The perception that girls mature early has obvious psychosocial consequences: they are treated as more mature and certainly behave in a more mature fashion. The latter is not, I suspect, just a result of conditioning. Testosterone is a difficult hormone to live with, and the first exposure can be very disturbing: I have even seen one 19 year-old boy prepubertal due to treatment of a craniopharyngioma rendered psychotic by the relatively small dose of testosterone I prescribed for him. Boys in early puberty become very active and easily distracted; they are much less diligent than girls, less compliant and often less successful. Thus female players in school orchestras outnumber males by at least 3 to 1. The reverse is seen later in many walks of life and I do not believe this just to be due to prejudice or the obvious biological problem of women pursuing demanding careers. When harnessed, testosterone gives drive to males which females lack and many females simply do not wish to compete in a male environment – *vive la différence.*

Early puberty

The symptoms which give rise to concern are breast development, penile or clitoral enlargement, axillary hair, pubic hair, acne and apocrine sweat when they would not be expected, that is before the age of 8 years in a girl and before the age of 9 years in a boy (see Fig. 3.7). The first task is to decide whether the consonance of the physical findings (secondary sexual characteristics, growth, bone maturity, etc) indicates the onset of true puberty (Fig. 3.9). Because girls with signs of early puberty outnumber boys in clinical practice by about 10 to 1 and because I have yet to see or hear of a boy with truly idiopathic central precocious puberty, signs of early pubertal development in boys are a much greater cause for concern.

Early breast development

Many infants are born with breast development because of exposure to maternal estrogen in utero but this soon subsides. In some girls it either persists or recurs during the early months or years of life, certainly before the age of 3 years. Such development is usually associated with isolated ovarian cyst development easily seen on pelvic ultrasound and attributable to premature but isolated pulsatile FSH secretion (Fig. 3.10). This condition is called *premature thelarche.* Uterine dimensions are appropriate for age, there is no endometrial echo and vaginal bleeding rarely if ever occurs. Growth continues at a normal rate and the bone age is appropriate for age. There are no other signs of puberty, such as pubic hair.

This is a benign condition. It needs no investigation beyond clinical examination, growth assessment and (if possible) pelvic ultrasonography. It needs no treatment. The natural history is for the condition to continue largely unchanged, although sometimes the breast development waxes and wanes in parallel to ovarian cyst size, until true puberty occurs. As long as growth continues at a normal rate, and no other signs of puberty appear, the patient needs only reassurance that all is well.

Breast development is, of course, the earliest sign of female puberty so

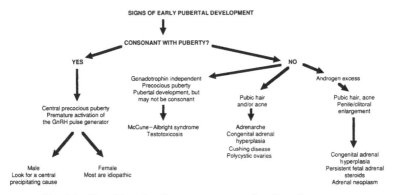

Fig. 3.9. Algorithm for the management of early puberty

the appearance of pubic hair, an increased growth velocity or a change in uterine dimensions requires the management of precocious puberty (p. 72).

Unfortunately, some girls cannot be categorized as falling into the class of either premature thelarche or precocious puberty because they have features of both. We call this condition *thelarche variant* and it presents with isolated breast development, increased stature, advanced bone age, a small uterus and ovarian morphology which is typical of neither premature thelarche nor precocious puberty (Fig. 3.11). The natural history of this condition, which seems also to be due to isolated pulsatile FSH secretion, is benign and growth prognosis is not compromised. It has been described as a benign variant of precocious puberty with a good prognosis by workers in Paris, and it needs no treatment unless the breast development is an embarrassment in which case cyproterone acetate is the first line of treatment to employ.

Isolated breast development in an older girl is usually the first sign of her puberty, in which case she will be increasing her growth rate. If she is not doing so, however, breast development may be a sign of (usually compensated) hypothyroidism and thyroid function should be assessed (Chapter 4). The reason why primary hypothyroidism causes breast development is that thyrotrophin releasing hormone (TRH) stimulates not only TSH but also prolactin and FSH. A girl may therefore exhibit ovarian cyst development and estradiol secretion without entering true puberty. The counterpart in a boy is enlargement of the testes without changes in genital appearance and, usually, short stature secondary to longstanding hypothyroidism.

Gynaecomastia in boys of pubertal age is extremely common. Indeed, some breast development always occurs in male puberty, even if it only

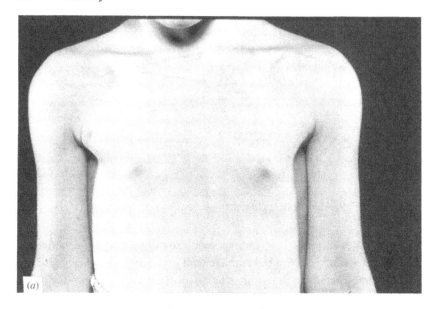

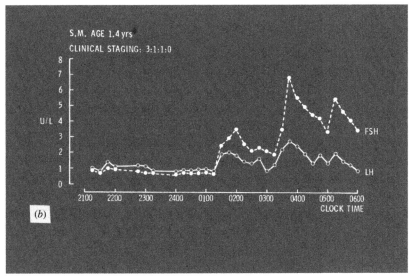

Fig. 3.10. Premature thelarche: (*a*) clinical appearance, (*b*) gonado-trophin profile; note FSH concentration at night greater than LH.

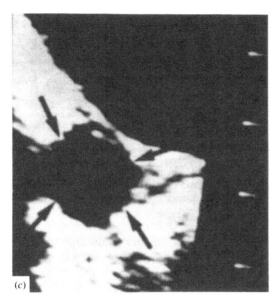

Fig. 3.10. Premature thelarche: (c) ultrasound findings; note a single large ovarian follicle/cyst.

manifests as some breast tenderness; it is, in fact, difficult to explain why all boys do not acquire marked breast development since the levels of circulating estrogen are certainly as high as those seen in a girl in early puberty. It presumably has to do with the balance between the levels of androgens and estrogens because, in the majority of instances, pubertal breast development subsides in boys as their puberty progresses. It persists in girls because the levels of androgens remain low; if they do not do so for any reason, breast development may be very slight.

In boys in whom there is a lack of testosterone secretion for any reason (e.g. biosynthetic defects or testicular abnormalities such as dysgenetic testes or Klinefelter syndrome), gynaecomastia will increase and may present as the primary complaint. The measurement of concentrations of LH and FSH, which should be low in any normal male, and of testosterone, which may be low in an afternoon clinic in a normal male, and especially low at any time of day in a boy in early puberty, will usually exclude pathology and karyotype examination is not usually indicated. In the vast majority of patients there is no endocrine abnormality to account for gyanecomastia which may be regarded as a transient part of normal puberty.

For a normally developed boy who has normal testicular function, large female-type breasts can be a source of great anxiety and embarrassment.

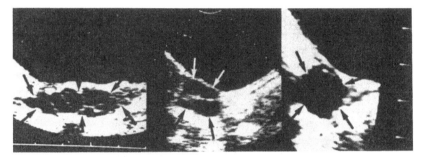

Fig. 3.11. Thelarche variant: ultrasound ovarian appearances contrasted with those of premature thelarche (RH panel), where a single large cyst occurs, and precocious puberty (LH panel) with a multicystic appearance.

They will not go away with medical therapy (additional testosterone) or with weight loss (although this may improve the cosmetic appearance of a fat boy) and I do not hesitate to refer such a boy for subareolar mastectomy, which has very satisfactory results. Most urologists are used to performing such operations on males treated with estrogens or castration for carcinoma of the prostate.

Breast development in an infant boy is rare but alarming. The child has to be investigated to exclude an exogenous source of estrogen (mother's contraceptive pills, for example), the presence of ovarian tissue (true hermaphroditism), a functioning adrenal or testicular tumour or another source of endogenous estrogen production which may be very difficult to discover.

Penile enlargement

This is a sign of androgen secretion which must originate in the testes or adrenal glands. If the testes are enlarged, especially if pubic hair is also present, the boy has precocious puberty (q.v.). If the testes are not enlarged, the adrenal source of androgen has to be determined; it is likely to be due to a functioning tumour or to congenital adrenal hyperplasia (see Chapter 5, page 109).

Clitoral enlargement

The clitoris can appear alarmingly large in the premature neonate because there is no fat in the labia majora. When this appears in the third trimester, the problem disappears. Sometimes, however, it fails to do so (Fig. 3.12),

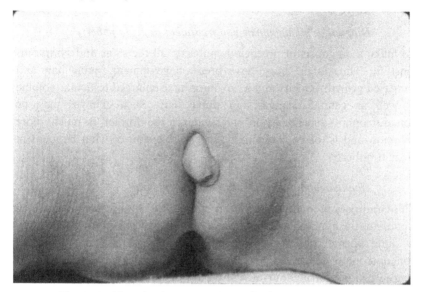

Fig. 3.12. Clitoral enlargement due to fetal adrenal androgens.

and sometimes the clitoris enlarges markedly after birth in the early postnatal period. My colleagues and I suspect that this is usually due to the persistent secretion of the androgens (DHA sulphate) from the fetal adrenal gland. As this involutes spontaneously, the clitoris usually becomes proportionate but embarrassing enlargement may persist necessitating surgery. In one patient, the clitoris, which had been reduced in infancy even though we had been unable to define the cause of its enlargement, grew again in middle childhood; another operation was required to reduce it during which a unilateral ovotestis was found.

When the clitoris grows abnormally after the newborn period, a source of endogenous androgen has to be suspected. This could be a virilizing tumour of the ovary, or of a dysgenetic testis, but is more likely to be due to an adrenal source of androgens (see Chapter 5).

Pubic hair, axillary hair, acne and apocrine sweat

These are all signs of androgen activity and are most frequently due to an adrenal source of androgens (e.g.adrenarche, congenital adrenal hyperplasia, Cushing syndrome or an adrenal tumour) in a boy or girl of prepubertal age. In a pubertal girl, particularly a tall one or a fat one, *polycystic ovarian syndrome* (page 79) is much more probable, although the other causes should be excluded.

Diagnosis, management and treatment of early puberty

To make a diagnosis of precocious puberty, all the signs and symptoms must fit. Thus a girl must have breast development, pubic hair and increased growth velocity and a boy must have enlarged testicular volume as well as genital changes and pubic hair. Such changes may be gonadotrophin dependent or independent; the former is much more common and is, of course, simply an early version of what happens in normal puberty.

Gonadotrophin dependent precocious puberty

This comprises premature activation of the GnRH pulse generator which stimulates the hypothalamo-pituitary–gonadal axis. This may be the onset of quite normal puberty or secondary to a cerebral cause. Proof of gonadotrophin dependency requires the measurement of LH and FSH concentrations throughout a 24 h period but the morphological (multicystic) appearance of the ovary on pelvic ultrasound is an important pointer (Fig. 3.3*b*). Stimulation of gonadotrophin concentrations with GnRH is useful in excluding gonadotrophin independent precocious puberty; in that condition there will be an inappropriately low response for the stage of puberty to such a stimulus.

Management of precocious puberty requires growth assessment (including pubertal staging), clinical examination (including neurological examination), visual field assessment to confrontation and fundoscopy, together with estimate of skeletal maturity. Where everything fits a consonant whole, and where there are no unusual signs or symptoms and the patient is female, pelvic ultrasonography will reveal multicystic ovaries (Fig. 3.3*b*) and an enlarging uterus (Fig. 3.4*b*), and no further investigations are required. If there is any doubt about neurological signs or symptoms, and always in a boy, imaging of the brain is required, preferably using nuclear magnetic resonance rather than computed tomography because the definition of MRI is greatly superior to even the most detailed CT. A cause must be found to explain precocious puberty in males. It is never 'idiopathic'.

Treatment

Where a cause has been found, it will be treated. In the case of a brain abnormality, the indication for any treatment should be neurological or neurosurgical: intervention will not improve the endocrine situation.

As far as the puberty is concerned, there has to be serious consideration of what is to be achieved by therapy. The adverse effects of precocious puberty are physical (being different from peers, menstruating at an inappropriate age, being unable to contain sexual drive, masturbation, etc) emotional, social and psychological. If the child is well adjusted in every way, there is probably no indication for treatment, especially if the progress of puberty is slow and there is not likely to be serious compromise of adult stature.

The growth problem (having a take-off of the pubertal component of growth at an insufficient height on the childhood curve) has hitherto been refractory to treatment. This was because the means to prolong or increase growth on the childhood curve was not available. The height prediction at diagnosis does not change with time and simply delaying puberty by therapy does not allow improvement in adult height because both the growth velocity and the rate of skeletal advance fell equally with the introduction of treatment. Thus the height–chronological age–bone age relation does not change.

With the ready availability of growth hormone treatment, this problem is beginning to be resolved: a child with precocious puberty, and a poor height prognosis through excessive advance of skeletal maturity, can be given medication to hold up puberty together with growth hormone to support and possibly accelerate growth along the childhood curve. The arrest of puberty will halt bone age maturation and growth hormone will improve height attained so that the height–chronological age–bone age equation moves in the right direction.

This is now regular in clinical practice but long term results are not yet available: final proof of the efficacy of this logical approach has to await the cessation of treatment and the attainment of final height. It is possible that it will prove very difficult to support growth for long enough to ameliorate the final height, although it has to be said that the prospects at present look rather encouraging, more encouraging in this sphere than in many of the current trials of the efficacy of growth hormone. The effect of GH on an ovary deprived of gonadotrophin control requires further elucidation. The use of GH is certainly associated with the ultrasound appearance of polycystic ovaries and these increase in size when gonadotrophin secretion is restored. Until this problem has been further researched, GH should not generally be used for this indication.

The pubertal process can be arrested at pituitary level through the use of gonadotrophin releasing hormone analogues, which occupy the GnRH receptors and prevent pulsatile gonadotrophin secretion. It is not necessary to ablate gonadotrophin secretion since the abolition of pulsatility is what is required. GnRH analogues are effective at halting puberty whether given intranasally, subcutaneously, or by depot injection. All the analogues

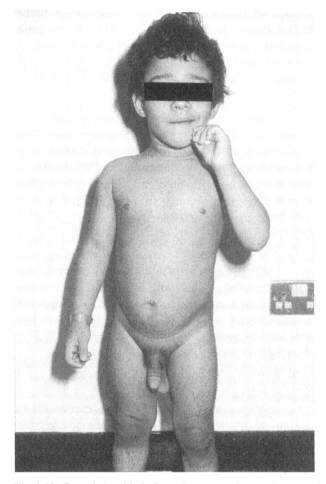

Fig. 3.13. Gonadotrophin independent precocious puberty in a 2 year-old boy.

available seem equally effective, so my preference is for a long-acting depot GnRH analogue which can be given at three- to four-weekly intervals (depending on the age of the patient and the stage of puberty) together in boys and possibly girls with daily subcutaneous injections of growth hormone, if the growth prognosis is too low when the growth velocity falls with the arrest of puberty and suppression of sex steroid secretion.

The introduction of this treatment sometimes provokes an estrogen withdrawal bleed; this can be prevented by the concomitant introduction of a progestagenic agent, such as cyproterone acetate or medroxy-

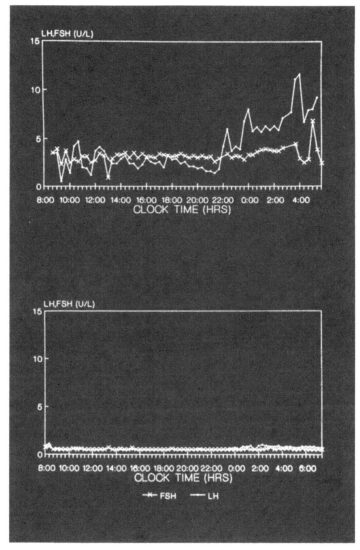

Fig. 3.13. Gonadotrophin independent precocious puberty in a 2 year-old boy: gonadotrophin profile (lower panel) contrasted with normal puberty (upper panel).

progesterone, which used to be the mainstays of treatment. If a bleed does occur with this combined treatment, it will be scanty, and of short duration, and it will not recur.

Gonadotrophin independent precocious puberty (GIPP)

The manifestations of GIPP, which is very rare, are identical to normal puberty except that the gonad matures independently of gonadotrophin stimulation for reasons which are not yet known. The criteria for the diagnosis are:

1. elevated testosterone/estradiol levels in the absence of gonadotrophin pulsatility;
2. blunted responsiveness to GnRH compared to age and stage of puberty;
3. no response to treatment with GnRH analogues.

In girls, the hallmark is the finding of one or more large ovarian cysts on ultrasound examination rather than the multicystic appearance typically secondary to nocturnal gonadotrophin pulsatility. This occurs most commonly in association with the skin pigmentation and bone abnormalities of the McCune–Albright syndrome. Other endocrine gland hyperactivity (thyroid, adrenal, pituitary) also occurs. The reason for this is probably to be found in the loss of the G (guanine nucleotide binding) proteins, one of which inhibits enzyme activity. Mutations within exon 8 of the $G_s\alpha$ gene are present in various tissues of patients with the McCune–Albright syndrome. These can lead to increased activity of the G_s protein which allows unregulated hormone secretion.

In boys, the name testotoxicosis has been attached to the autonomous secretion of testosterone; the clinical appearance can be very striking (Fig. 3.13). The aetiology of the condition is not known but it could well turn out to be attributed to a similar situation.

For boys or girls, treatment to suppress puberty has to be at gonadal level and is given as cyproterone acetate, medroxyprogesterone or an inhibitor of steroid biosynthesis (ketoconazole or testolactone) or peripheral action (e.g. flutamide for androgen excess).

Late puberty

When no signs of secondary sexual development are seen in a boy aged 14 years or a girl aged 13 years, thought is needed (Fig. 3.14). It is important to stress the adjective 'no'; if the testes have started to enlarge or there is

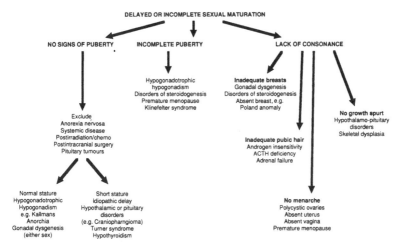

Fig. 3.14. Algorithm for the management of late puberty

the slightest sign of breast development, there is room for reassurance and a follow-up visit to ensure that puberty is progressing.

Even if there are no signs of puberty, the patient may yet enter puberty spontaneously but the chances of doing so diminish with time. The differential diagnosis is much more alarming in girls than in boys, and of more concern in patients of either sex if their height is not also proportionately small. Concern may also be expressed about a child who has incomplete puberty for any reason.

No signs of puberty

General physical examination and a careful history ought to give a clue to the presence of physical disease. Of the conditions shown at the bottom left of Fig. 3.14, eating disorders, asthma, Crohn's disease and pituitary adenomata are the major pitfalls for the unwary. Thinness is helpful in excluding most of the endocrine causes of late puberty.

When the patient is of normal stature, hypogonadotrophic hypogonadism is the major disorder to consider, and its differential from gonadal failure is easily determined by the estimation of LH and FSH concentrations. Where these are elevated, the problem is distal to the pituitary gland. If they are low, the patient may have a hypothalamo-pituitary problem or may have 'simple' delay of puberty: unfortunately, there is no way to distinguish these two entities except by awaiting the passage of time. Pointers can be gained from pelvic ultrasonography (the absence of multicystic change in a teenager is unusual) and from hormone profiles (there ought to be nocturnal pulsatile gonadotrophin secretion) but I have known both to mislead. Note that the measurement of sex steroid concentrations is a waste of time and money; they will be low.

It is possible to use the time needed to establish the diagnosis by instituting treatment to induce puberty. The maturational process will proceed in spite of this and the patient's own pubertal development will 'overtake' the therapy provided (see below).

If the patient is of short stature, the probability is that he or she has idiopathic delay of puberty but this does not mean that treatment may not be required for psychological reasons. The measurement of gonadotrophin concentrations will distinguish hypergonadotrophic hypogonadism from hypogonadotrophic hypogonadism: in a girl, the former is probably associated with short stature in the Turner syndrome. If the LH and FSH concentrations are high in a girl, a karyotype is useful. It is always worth excluding the diagnosis of hypothyroidism. If they are low, a measurement of serum prolactin concentration is a wise precaution to exclude the presence of a prolactinoma.

Since the differential diagnosis of hypogonadotrophic hypogonadism includes hypothalamo-pituitary disease, the threshold for performing an imaging procedure should be low but cannot (or should not) be performed on every patient with idiopathic delay. Indicators include a height prediction which is low or high for the family (i.e. a disproportionate bone age), and a growth velocity which is low even for the age and stage of puberty. If 5 cm/year is accepted as normal for a prepubertal 12 year old of either sex, this may be expected to fall in a child continuing to show no signs of puberty by 1 cm/year for every year that elapses so that, by the age of 17–18, growth will be at a standstill until sex steroids are introduced. (A similar rate of fall in growth velocity will also be seen in a patient on growth hormone therapy until sex steroids are secreted or introduced.) A normal lower limit of velocity may be taken as 1 cm/year less than these figures and I use such a yardstick to decrease my threshold for requesting an imaging procedure.

Incomplete puberty

Where the physical signs of puberty appear in a consonant fashion, they may 'get stuck' at any stage of maturity and reproductive capability is not acquired. Such a situation merges into the general problem of infertility because hypogonadotrophic hypogonadism may, for example, present to the paediatric endocrinologist as no, or partial, puberty or to the infertility clinic as ovulatory failure. The latter patients often get treated with oral estrogens in their late teens and then present with 'post-pill amenorrhoea', a misnomer for (treated) prepill amenorrhoea.

Puberty may also start but not be completed if there is a block in sex steroidogenesis. It may be possible with high gonadotrophic drive to force the production of sex steroids to a certain extent but full puberty may well not be achievable. Such a circumstance will be highlighted by a discrepancy between the concentrations of testosterone or estradiol and LH and FSH.

Lack of consonance (Fig. 3.14)

Particular clinical acumen is required to identify and diagnose a partial failure of one component of puberty, especially as the patient may well complain of a symptom not immediately referable to physical development.

As well as inadequate breast development, unequal breasts cause teenagers anxiety. This may be relatively slight and still be very worrying to the patient: it is often the result of a whole body asymmetry which has not been previously identified. Surgery is sometimes needed for breast reduction on one side or augmentation mammoplasty on the other, but neither procedure should be contemplated until puberty is as complete as it is going to be in the individual with or without treatment.

Inadequate pubic hair development points some serious diagnoses but it must be remembered that pubic hair in females is the result of adrenal androgen secretion. This will be diminished by any steroid medication which suppresses ACTH secretion. It is not easy to treat because of the side effects of androgens in girls (see below).

Polycystic ovarian disease is by far the commonest cause of delayed menarche. Polycystic ovaries (PCO) can be found on ultrasound (Fig. 3.15) in about one quarter of the female adult population and may, therefore, be regarded as a normal variant. They account for 87% of irregular menstrual cycles in unselected adult females. The incidence of polycystic ovaries is familial and they may be inherited from the father's or mother's side of the family. The gene or genes have not been identified but hyperandrogenemia and hyperinsulinemia are both powerful predisposing causes, as may be seen in girls with congenital adrenal hyperplasia and/or with tall stature.

The polycystic ovarian (Stein–Leventhal) *syndrome* (polycystic ovaries, oligomenorrhoea, hirsutism and obesity) does not occur in every patient with PCO but there is clearly some question of chicken and egg between causes and consequences of PCO which is important for the patient. The

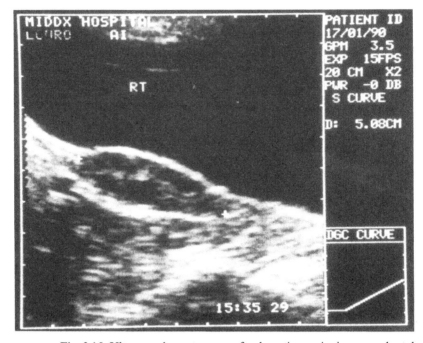

Fig. 3.15. Ultrasound appearances of polycystic ovaries in a prepubertal girl.

consequences of PCO syndrome can be extremely worrying to a teenager and have to be treated just as in the adult with antiandrogen and cyclical estrogen (see Chapter 10).

In general, there is no lack of estrogenization in a patient with PCO but vaginal bleeding does not occur unless there is sufficient waxing and waning of estradiol concentrations to provoke an estrogen withdrawal bleed from the uterus. This may be not only delayed, a symptom which may be sufficiently distressing to require treatment in its own right, but also become irregular in frequency and amount. In either case there is a good argument for instituting cycle control medication, effectively the birth control pill.

The easiest problem to miss, but the one which perhaps has the longest term adverse consequences, is the lack of a growth spurt. The contribution of the pubertal growth spurt to final height is about 25 cm and lack of GH or sex steroids causes irrevocable loss of about half of this total. Loss of sex steroid secretion is usually obvious (it is what this chapter is about) but the inability to augment pulsatile GH secretion in response to sex steroids is difficult to identify if it is unexpected.

Table 3.1. *Duration of puberty* (*Years taken to progress from stage 2 to 5*)

Centiles*	3%	50%	97%
Breasts/genitalia			
Girls	1.5	4.0	9.0*
Boys	1.9	3.1	4.7
Pubic hair			
Girls	1.4	2.5	3.1
Boys	2.4	3.2	4.2

* 3% of girls progress from Breast stage 2 to 5 in 1.5 years, 50% will have done so over 4.0 years. (Some girls do not acquire Breast stage 5 until pregnancy, which is why the 97th centile for stage 5 is apparently so protracted.)

Particular traps await the patient who has had cranial irradiation (e.g. for leukemia) but idiopathic GH deficiency may present at this age as a result of a very minor degree of pituitary hypoplasia. The idea that this results in an all-or-nothing syndrome is quite wrong: if growth velocity results from the concentration of peaks of GH (amplitude modulation), the amount of GH secreted must increase as the size of the child increases. It may fail to do so at any age, including puberty, and the patient will then need GH replacement treatment. In puberty, the identification of this problem is particularly important because the epiphyses of the untreated patient will fuse before adequate growth has occurred.

Skeletal dysplasias are a special cause of the failure of pubertal growth. For whatever reason, and the cause is not known, no patient with a skeletal dysplasia ever increases his or her growth rate at puberty, and the result is the increased disproportion seen in adult patients with, say, hypo-chondroplasia. The remedy for this situation may be GH treatment but the issue is *sub judice* at the moment. GH should *not* be used indiscriminately in the puberty years because it shortens the duration of the process and may, therefore, frustrate the object of therapy.

Treatment (For details, see Chapter 10 (page 171)

When puberty needs to be induced, or breast or genitalia size increased, sex steroids will be employed but it is important to remember the time scale of normal development (Table 3.1) and to try not to exceed it. In particular, the temptation to go more rapidly in the older patient must be resisted if possible. In boys, the effects of testosterone can be very alarming. In girls, a shortened puberty caused by the use of excessive doses of estrogen results in inadequate breast growth (with excessive brown nipple development) and, more importantly, inadequate uterine development which may frustrate a later attempt at embryo transfer for anovulatory infertility.

When pubic hair is inadequate in a girl, she needs androgens but these are difficult to give without inducing unwanted side effects, especially male pattern baldness and voice changes. Oral testosterone undecanoate can be quite useful here; in a male patient, this medication is not useful because of the conversion to dihydrotestosterone but this conversion to a relatively weak androgen can be helpful for girls. Anabolic steroids may also be used.

The indications for using GH treatment in puberty are few but, as indicated, important. For patients with a normal skeleton, 15 units/m²/week is a dose sufficient to promote growth in the GH deficient patient but probably insufficient greatly to accelerate puberty. For patients with an abnormal skeleton (skeletal dysplasia, Turner syndrome, etc), a bigger dose may be required, just how big in the range 20–40 IU/m²/week is not established.

For boys with 'simple' or 'constitutional' delay of puberty, sex steroids are very useful. These may be given as anabolic steroids in low dose to promote growth or as testosterone to accelerate both growth and puberty. Details of these treatments are to be found in Chapter 10 (page 172).

4

The thyroid gland

Clinical physiology

The thyroid gland forms in the third week of gestation as an endodermal proliferation from the pharyngeal gut to which it remains attached by the thyroglossal duct. This subsequently fragments and disappears, although remnants may cause problems as thyroglossal cysts. The thyroid gland is made up of lobules composed of follicles. Their task is to synthesize, iodinate and store thyroglobulin and subsequently to reabsorb it, degrade the protein and release the hormones.

The steps in synthesis and release include:

1. iodide trapping by the thyroid gland;
2. synthesis of thyroglobulin in the follicular cells;
3. organification of trapped iodide as iodotyrosines;
4. coupling of the iodotyrosines to form iodothyronines;
5. storage of iodothyronines in extracellular colloid;
6. invagination and formation of intracellular colloid droplets;
7. hydrolysis of thyroglobulin to release iodotyrosines, T3 and T4;
8. deiodination of the iodotyrosines and recirculation of the iodide; release of the T3 and T4 into the circulation.

Some thyroglobulin escapes degradation and reaches the circulation through thyroid lymphatics in association with iodothyronines. Circulating thyroglobulin levels are high in the neonate and decrease in infancy and childhood. Concentrations increase when the thyroid gland is hyperactive, including after TSH administration; they decrease during thyroxine administration.

The thyroid gland is the sole source of T4. 70–90 % of the T3 or reverse

T3 in blood is derived from the monodeiodination of T4 by peripheral tissues. T3 (monodeiodination of the β- or outer hydroxyl ring of T4) has three to four times the metabolic potency of T4. Monodeiodination of the inner or α-hydroxyl ring of T4 produces reverse or rT3, which is inactive in postnatal life, although it may serve a fetal purpose.

T4 is bound in plasma by thyroxine binding globulin (TBG). Albumin and TBG seem about equally important for the carriage of T3. Free T4 and T3 levels account for approximately 0.03 and 0.30% of total values, absolute levels being about 20 and 2 pmol/l respectively.

The hormones are excreted in the urine and faeces in free and conjugated forms.

Regulation of thyroid function

TSH controls expression of the thyroglobulin gene and also modulates most of the synthetic and secretory processes outlined above. TSH is itself stimulated by TRH secretion from the hypothalamus and is inhibited by somatostatin and dopamine. TRH release is stimulated by body cooling. Monodeiodination of T4 in the pituitary yields T3 which exerts negative feedback at the pituitary level by inhibiting TSH release.

Thyroid hormone effects

Thyroid hormones penetrate cell membranes and bind to a specific nuclear receptor. T3 binds to the nuclear receptor with ten times the affinity of T4 and also binds to plasma membrane and mitochondrial receptors, though for what purpose is not clear. The major effects of thyroid hormones are mediated via the nuclear T3 receptors modulating gene transcription and synthesis of mRNA and cytoplasmic proteins. T3 also stimulates mitochondrial activity and, through these various sites of action, modulates many physiological processes.

These include thermogenesis, water and ion transport, lipid and amino acid substrate turnover and growth factor production and action. Thyroid hormones also potentiate the actions of catecholamines by increasing β-adrenergic receptor binding and postreceptor responsiveness. This is why the tachycardia, tremor and lid-lag of hyperthyroidism can be helped by β-receptor blocking agents such as propranolol.

Fetal and neonatal thyroid function

The fetal pituitary–thyroid axis functions independently of the maternal system. The placenta is impermeable to TSH and only small amounts of maternal T4 and T3 cross to the fetus. The placenta also inactivates maternal thyroid hormones, so the fetus largely functions on its own. Thyroid gland activity increases in the second and third trimesters and clearly has important and widespread functions in the development of the central nervous system.

Tests of thyroid function

The carriage of thyroid hormones by plasma proteins has already been mentioned. Where there are abnormalities in the concentration of the binding proteins, total concentration of thyroid hormones may appear abnormal, even though free hormone concentrations are unaffected. For this reason, indices of thyroid function were introduced (indirect ways of determining free hormone concentrations before assays were adequately sensitive to measure the very low concentrations accurately), but these have been superseded by direct free hormone assays.

It is also possible to measure TBG concentrations. This can be important in the context of neonatal screening for levels of T4 because the prevalence of TBG deficiency or insufficiency varies from 1 in 5000 to 1 in 10000 newborns, which is close to the incidence of congenital hypothyroidism. Total T4 levels will be low in affected individuals but they are euthyroid, have normal TSH concentrations, normal responses to TRH and do not need treatment. Conversely, subjects with increased levels of TBG have increased serum T4 concentrations with normal free T4 and TSH concentrations and are thus euthyroid.

For the majority of patients these esoterica are unimportant but the clinician needs to be aware of the pitfalls if he is receiving results of thyroid function tests. He would be wise in the first instance to stick to measurements of total T4 and TSH.

Where T4 is low, the TSH concentration in a sensitive assay may be above the normal range (primary hypothyroidism), below it (secondary hypothyroidism) or normal. In the third case, there may be tertiary hypothyroidism or there may be a carrier protein problem which assays for TBG and free hormone concentrations will sort out.

Where T4 is high, the TSH concentration in a sensitive assay may be low (hyperthyroidism) or normal in which case the further assays are required.

Table 4.1. *Causes of hypothyroidism*

Congenital disorders
Primary disease
– dysgenetic gland
– inborn error of hormonogenesis
Secondary disease
– TSH deficiency, isolated or multiple defect
Transient disorders
Acquired disorders
Primary disease
– iodine deficiency
– goitrogens
– autoimmune thyroiditis
– postirradiation and/or chemotherapy
Secondary disease
– TSH deficiency
Tertiary disease
– TRH deficiency

Hypothyroidism

The causes of hypothyroidism in childhood are shown in Table 4.1. The *sine qua non* of making a diagnosis is to demonstrate that the concentrations of thyroid hormones are below the normal range.

In primary hypothyroidism, the gland itself is in trouble so the serum TSH concentration will be raised and the TSH response to injected TRH will be exaggerated (see Chapter 10).

By secondary hypothyroidism is meant low T4 and T3 levels secondary to a pituitary deficiency of TSH. In this situation, TSH levels will be low and the response to TRH negligible.

In hypothalamic disease, there is deficiency of TRH: the basal TSH concentration will be low and it will rise and continue rising after an injection of TRH as the releasable TSH emerges from the understimulated pituitary gland.

Because TRH is a powerful stimulator of prolactin, concentrations of this hormone are raised in primary thyroid disease, abnormally low in pituitary disease and intermediately raised in any situation where the secretory path of dopamine from the hypothalamus to the pituitary is interrupted. Values of its concentration are thus extremely useful in clinical practice. Very high concentrations are indicative of a pituitary tumour (prolactinoma).

As mentioned in Chapter 3, TRH also stimulates FSH secretion. In a hypothyroid girl, this manifests as breast enlargement secondary to ovarian cyst formation. In a hypothyroid boy, the testicular volume is often considerably larger than it should be for the other signs of puberty. In patients of both sexes, the skeletal maturity will be surprisingly delayed for the apparent stage of puberty. Indeed, a bone age–chronological age discrepancy of more than 3 years in any patient always points the need for thyroid function tests.

Congenital hypothyroidism

1 in 4000 infants are born with congenital hypothyroidism, and few of them manifest clinical evidence of T4 deficiency. Detection based on signs and symptoms, such as an umbilical hernia, large tongue, constipation, feeding problems, lethargy, respiratory problems, jaundice or hoarse cry (listed here in descending order of prevalence) will usually be delayed 6–12 weeks or longer, which is why neonatal screening programmes were introduced.

Without treatment, there is progressive accumulation of soft tissue myxedema leading to a large tongue, difficulty in swallowing, hoarse cry (myxedema of the vocal cords) and hypotonia. Cretinoid facies and growth failure become progressively more obvious over the first year of life.

Screening infant blood samples for T4 and/or TSH concentrations is now widespread and in most hypothyroid infants there are low values of T4 and elevated TSH concentrations. However 10–20 % of infants with hypothyroidism have T4 values in the low–normal range so the screening cut-off has to be rather high in a T4 based programme, and the recall rate of infants for retesting is correspondingly high. 10 % of hypothyroid infants have a TSH value < 50 mIU/l and a few have < 20 mIU/l with a delayed postnatal rise to the hypothyroid range. As infants with TSH and TRH deficiencies are likely to be missed by any screening programme, the index of clinical suspicion needs to be maintained.

Most infants with congenital hypothyroidism have thyroid dysgenesis but they may have ectopic thyroid tissue (which may fail at a later age) and they may have a defect of thyroid hormone synthesis. I take the view that affected children will need replacement treatment whatever the result, and cannot see much point in the routine scanning of such patients.

Congenital TRH or TSH deficiencies are much less common than congenital primary disease. Isolated deficiencies have to be diagnosed clinically, but secondary or tertiary hypothyroidism may be just one component of panhypopituitarism which is likely to present with hypo-glycemia due to GH and/or ACTH deficiencies, with micropenis due to LH deficiency or with conjugated hyperbilirubinemia due to cortisol deficiency which may be secondary to ACTH deficiency. Many such infants have midline cranial defects which may or may not be immediately obvious (e.g. cleft palate).

Transient thyroid dysfunction

Serum T4 concentrations increase with gestational age so all premature neonates have some degree of transient hypothyroxinemia. This causes no ill effects, will correct itself with time, and needs no treatment. Premature babies are also relatively inefficient at the conversion of T4 to T3, so low levels of T3 may be found in otherwise well infants. This should not cause alarm if the T4 and TSH concentrations are within the normal range.

Transient primary hypothyroidism certainly does exist and it cannot be distinguished from the permanent condition. Accordingly, all babies with low T4 concentrations and high TSH values should be treated. At a later date (I usually wait until the third year of life), the dose of thyroxine administered should be allowed to fall below replacement level to determine its continuing need by a rising TSH concentration. An alternative strategy is to convert the child to T3 treatment for 4 weeks, to discontinue the treatment for a week and then to measure T4 and TSH levels and perform a TRH test. T4 treatment should be restored while awaiting results.

Transient hyperthyrotropinemia (high TSH with normal T4) has emerged as a condition because of neonatal screening programmes. This condition does not require treatment but it needs follow-up to exclude a disorder such as an ectopic thyroid gland or dyshormonogenesis. The TSH concentration generally falls spontaneously over a period of 3–6 months.

Acquired hypothyroidism

This may occur at any age and the onset is gradual. It may be extremely hard to diagnose clinically (even with knowledge of the biochemical results) so a high index of suspicion should be maintained by all clinicians. The most obvious symptom is slowing of growth velocity leading to short stature. Gain in weight and fat is usually modest but a disproportion between weight and height gain may cause comment. The secretion of FSH may lead to isolated breast development without an increase in height velocity or to testicular enlargement without signs of androgen secretion. Pubertal delay or arrest can be another presentation.

Obvious signs of classical hypothyroidism and myxedema, including the mental slowness, are very slow to develop and they are rare in a prepubertal child, however severe the biochemical disorder. This is presumably simply a matter of time; adult patients with obvious signs have simply been hypothyroid for longer. Hypothyroid children actually do rather well at school because they are quiet, slow, peaceful, happy and compliant. They have characteristically slow tendon reflex contraction and very slow relaxation, but this may be the only clear physical finding.

Numerically, in the world, iodine deficiency must still rate as the commonest cause of thyroid dysfunction and this state is particularly dangerous to the fetus which may well be born not only with a goitre but also with a serious neurological developmental handicap. Iodine deficiency can also be caused by goitrogens introduced in medications or food. Epidemiologically, this is an important state to eliminate by public health measures, and these have been effective in removing this cause of hypothyroidism in most of Western Europe and the United States. Pockets of endemic cretinism do remain in these areas, however, and are also seen in Eastern Europe, South America and elsewhere.

Iodine supplementation of food will eliminate the problem and will reduce the incidence of hypothyroidism and of thyroid carcinoma caused by longstanding borderline hypothyroidism and high TSH values. The disadvantage of widespread increase in iodine intake is an increase in the incidence of hyperthyroidism. I believe that this is probably the reason why thyrotoxicosis seems to be commoner amongst children with autoimmune thyroid disease in North America as compared to Western Europe.

In non-endemic goitre areas, autoimmune thyroiditis is by far the commonest cause of acquired hypothyroidism. Autoimmune thyroiditis may present clinically as thyrotoxicosis or as frank hypothyroidism, but mostly does so with a small goitre, a euthyroid state and compensated hypothyroidism (T4 in the low normal range with elevated TSH). The condition runs in families, presents in girls rather than boys, and may be associated with other autoimmune conditions such as diabetes mellitus, Addison disease, hypoparathyroidism, chronic mucocutaneous candidiasis, etc. Thyroid disorders in general, but autoimmune thyroid disease in particular, are associated with a number of other syndromes, such as those described by Down, Turner and Noonan. Since these conditions present with short stature, exclusion of a thyroid deficit should be routine, especially in Down and Noonan syndrome where mental retardation may also be a problem.

Most clinicians will be aware that the disease may present with short stature and a retarded bone age. As has already been mentioned, the presentation with isolated breast development or large testes is quite common and a low growth velocity in the face of these signs of puberty calls for a test of thyroid function long before short stature becomes an issue.

Many types of antibody have been described in association with autoimmune thyroiditis; antithyroglobulin and antimicrosomal antibodies are the most useful in clinical practice. They may be found in subjects who still have normal thyroid function but it should be the rule to take blood for antibody screening and thyroid function tests from every first-degree relative of a patient with autoimmune thyroiditis.

Hypothyroidism due to a dysgenetic gland or to a defect of thyroid hormone biosynthesis may well not present until later in childhood or at puberty. Only a high level of clinical acumen (or a blunderbuss approach to biochemical investigation) will prevent a late diagnosis.

Primary hypothyroidism has emerged as one of the commoner sequelae of the treatment of childhood cancers. Spinal irradiation inevitably includes the thyroid gland in its field and chemotherapy is additive in increasing the risk of thyroid dysfunction. Because children who have had one cancer are at risk from developing another, because irradiation is a predisposing cause of thyroid cancer, and because a persistently raised TSH concentration is also a risk factor for thyroid carcinoma, a careful and prospective watch should be kept on the T4 and TSH levels in patients who have had irradiation and /or chemotherapy. A raised TSH concentration should be treated with thyroxine without delay.

Hypothyroidism secondary to TSH deficiency is important to suspect because it will probably be missed on a neonatal thyroid screen. Isolated TSH deficiency is very rare; TSH deficiency is not so rare when combined with other pituitary deficiencies, especially of GH and gonadotrophins. TRH deficiency is probably commoner than TSH deficiency, especially in children with a hypothalamic cause of GH insufficiency, which is probably the majority of such children. It should be a matter of routine to watch the thyroid function of any child with hypopituitarism and to be especially vigilant when such a child is exposed to the stress of treatment with, say, growth hormone.

Treatment

In principle, the treatment of hypothyroidism, congenital or acquired, is simple: the dose of thyroxine is 100 μg/m^2/24 h given as a single oral preparation, and this applies throughout life.

There is dispute about monitoring treatment. After the introduction of thyroxine medication, it is not clear how quickly the TSH concentration falls at any age and it may be a function not only of age but also of the duration of its previous elevation. It is not worth titrating the initial dose against the fall of TSH for this reason. To do so also puts the patient at risk of overdose – and the effects of hyperthyroidism are probably more deleterious than those of hypothyroidism.

After treatment has been established, some physicians routinely measure T4 and TSH concentrations, but they have a problem justifying the former because the concentration varies in relation to the dose administered and the time when it was taken. Thyroxine tolerance tests are certainly not available for every individual patient!

TSH can be useful to show that a low dose has been prescribed but this should not have been allowed to happen and will anyway be spotted by growth assessment. I find TSH measurement useful only to judge compliance: if an adolescent has a normal T4 concentration and an elevated TSH in the out-patient clinic, it can be reasonably assumed that he took his medication that day because he was visiting the doctor but did not do so regularly. In practice, I do not perform routine thyroid function tests on treated hypothyroid patients unless they are not growing and developing as I expect or unless I suspect non-compliance.

In adult and older child patients it is probably worth starting with one-quarter of the full replacement dose for one week, then one-half for one week and so on. If there is any doubt about multiple pituitary hormone deficiency, it is sensible to cover the introduction of thyroxine in the older patient with glucocorticoid replacement unless or until the necessity for this has been excluded, but this is not needed in most infants and young children.

The real problem with treatment of hypothyroidism, particularly if it has been of longstanding, is that the hypothyroid child is comfortable to live with. He, or probably she, is quiet and biddable, compliant, studious and academically successful; give him thyroxine and he becomes impossible in every way. He is hyperactive, lacks concentration, fails at school, cannot sleep and so on; his parents much prefer his old self and either they, or he, may withold medication because of this. Parents and children must be warned of this effect, which has nothing to do with excessive dosage. The situation settles down with time but it may be 12–18 months before it does so – and parents may still mourn the hypothyroid child they no longer have.

The outcome of treatment of congenital hypothyroidism indicates that early thyroxine replacement has led to a marked reduction in the IQ deficit associated with the condition before screening. Complete restoration of performance does not seem to be possible, however, and a deficit of 5–10 IQ points is probably inevitable as a result of prenatal thyroxine deficiency. Thus 10% of hypothyroid children have an IQ less than 2sd below the population mean compared to 2% of controls. Replacement doses which give T4 levels which are persistently raised are definitely not in the patient's interest. Hyperthyroidism is very destructive (see below) and this is a good reason for not pursuing the goal of total TSH suppression on therapy.

Severe prenatal hypothyroidism leaves some special psychomotor deficits: parents complain about a lack of hand–eye coordination, which leads to poor writing skills. Mathematics seems to present particular difficulties to these children. Nevertheless, I know of one (reconfirmed) hypothyroid child who won scholarships to St Paul's and Oxford, so the handicap of what was certainly severe prenatal hypothyroidism may vary considerably from case to case. There seems to be no good evidence that the age at start of treatment has a major influence on outcome if that age is less than 50 days. There are few data on the effect of quality of treatment on outcome, probably because there is insufficient variation in that parameter. All evidence points to the fact that it is best to diagnose hypothyroidism as soon as possible and to treat it properly at any age.

Hyperthyroidism

The commonest cause of an overactive thyroid gland is that it is responding to thyroid stimulating immunoglobulins (TSI) of whatever type. When thyrotoxicosis is associated with eye manifestations, the term Graves' disease has been attached. Autonomous functioning thyroid nodules are very uncommon in children. Hyperthyroidism may also be due to autonomous TSH production from the pituitary thyrotroph or from pituitary tumours. It has also been attributed to a resistance to the feedback effect of T3 on TSH release.

Autoimmune hyperthyroidism

Thyrotoxicosis may present at any age but there is a sharp increase in the peripubertal years. Girls are affected 6–8 times more frequently than boys and a high proportion of patients have a family history of autoimmune thyroid disease. For this reason, the first degree relatives of a patient with thyrotoxicosis need thyroid function tests and antibody screening.

The clinical onset may be abrupt or insidious. Patients may present with school problems (lack of concentration, hyperactivity), tall stature, weight loss in spite of an increased appetite and the effects of increased β-adrenergic receptor binding and postreceptor responsiveness (tachycardia, tremor and lid lag). I have seen two children precipitated into cardiac failure by thyrotoxicosis, so the disease needs taking seriously. It is extremely destructive of school performance.

The infiltration of the orbit with mucopolysaccharides, lymphocytes and edema leads to exophthalmos, ophthalmoplegia and chemosis of the conjuctivae. Advanced eye disease is rare in children, but I have had to resort to tarsorrhaphy in one case, and I would not hesitate to seek the opinion of an expert in this complication of thyrotoxicosis because the treatment of the hyperthyroidism has little effect on the progression of the eye condition.

The biochemical hallmarks of this condition are a raised T4 concentration and a TSH concentration which is suppressed below the normal range. In cases of doubt, the T3 concentration can be measured as well as free hormone concentrations. A TRH test will show no TSH response.

Treatment

Treatment requires the administration of carbimazole or propylthiouracil in adequate doses (see chapter 10). Propranolol can be useful in the management of the acute situation. It is once the thyroid hormone concentrations have come under control that there is dispute about management. Thyrotoxicosis will remit at a rate of about 10 % per annum. The drugs have side effects. The disease is a nuisance.

My view is that children who have not remitted within 6–12 months may have to wait a long time to do so and that they suffer greatly in the waiting. I therefore favour instituting a definitive management strategy which means radioactive iodine or thyroidectomy.

Some parents are unwilling to go along with this (although those who decide to opt for a definitive treatment later nearly always regret that they had not done so earlier) and, in this situation or if there are problems of compliance, I favour a block-replacement regimen. This means using moderate doses of carbimazole or propylthiouracil together with thyroxine replacement in the usual dosage (100 $\mu g/m^2/24$ h). What is not useful is to try to titrate the dose of carbimazole to the T4 level; this means endless and frequent visits to the hospital and is very disruptive. Also, if the TSH concentration starts to rise, the goitre may enlarge and the hyperthyroid state be exacerbated.

The choice between surgery and radioactive iodine is difficult. On the one hand, the number of surgeons practised in thyroid surgery is falling and the operation is not without its hazards (hypoparathyroidism being the worst – and this can occur even if a competent surgeon has identified the parathyroid glands and left them well alone) but, on the other, one feels reluctant to administer radioactive substances to children, and an increased risk of cancer is a real concern. One thing is certain which is that hypothyroidism is the inevitable consequence of definitive treatment and a common occurrence with the passage of time in these patients anyway.

I work with a very competent thyroid surgeon so my own preference is towards surgery for definitive management. I treat the patient medically for about 6–9 months and then he operates on the euthyroid patient. We do not use preoperative iodine and we perform a total thyroidectomy. This is because the danger of relapse in a glandular remnant is considerable and reoperating is hazardous; it is very difficult to judge the necessary extent of a partial resection. Many paediatric endocrinologists, particularly in North America, favour radioactive iodine. All would agree that this is a disorder which needs taking seriously and needs definitive management.

Neonatal thyrotoxicosis

Thyrotoxicosis in pregnancy is rare, presumably because thyrotoxic ladies do not easily get pregnant. In thyrotoxic women who do get pregnant, the baby is affected by the passive transfer of maternal antibodies in about 1 in 70 instances, so neonatal thyrotoxicosis is very unusual.

An affected baby is irritable, flushed and tachycardic to the point of cardiac failure. Weight gain is poor. The baby has a goitre and exophthalmos and some may be extremely ill. Others may simply manifest some increase in T4, T3 and free hormone levels.

This condition is self-limiting; the half-life of maternally acquired antibodies is 12 days, so the disease subsides over 3–12 weeks. Treatment is symptomatic using sedatives and cardiac support as indicated. In severely ill babies, iodide is the first line of therapy and should be followed by antithyroid medication which can be increased if an adequate response is not quickly observed. Treatment must be carefully monitored by measuring TSH concentrations and should be progressively withdrawn once these start to rise.

Thyroid swellings

Thyroid neoplasia

A solitary thyroid mass of a consistency different from that of the rest of the thyroid gland suggests neoplasia, and the prevalence of malignancy is 15–20 %. Such nodules are very unusual in children. External irradiation has been shown to predispose to malignant change, especially when this is combined with chronic TSH drive from primary hypothyroidism.

Tumours of the follicular epithelium include follicular adenomata and papillary, follicular or anaplastic carcinomata. Tumours of non-follicular origin include medullary carcinoma, metastatic tumours, lymphoma and teratoma. They are all very rare in children except benign adenomata or cystic lesions.

Where there is any doubt on ultrasound or radioiodine uptake about the nature of a thyroid lump, a needle biopsy and cytology is the way to proceed. A functioning nodule is rarely malignant. Needle biopsy and cytology are much more frequently used in adult endocrine practice than in paediatric practice and the patient should be sent to a properly equipped clinic if possible.

Medullary thyroid carcinoma (MTC) is part of the neuroectodermal multiple endocrine neoplasia spectrum (MEN II, to be contrasted with MEN I, which comprises parathyroid, pituitary and pancreatic tumours). In MEN IIa, medullary carcinoma occurs with phaeochromocytoma and hyperparathyroidism, in MEN IIb with phaeochromocytoma and mucosal neuromata (bumpy lips). MTC is associated with increased secretion of calcitonin which can be provoked by intravenous calcitonin or pentagastrin in asymptomatic children of affected parents thus allowing thyroidectomy before the MTC is more than a few mm in size. Such tests should be performed biennially on children of affected families.

In general, cold nodules should be removed surgically unless cytology obviates the need. Frozen section will indicate the necessity to proceed to thyroidectomy and this is usually the end of the treatment, radiotherapy prophylaxis not being of proven benefit. After such treatment, continuous suppression of TSH with adequate thyroxine replacement is essential to avoid stimulation of residual tumour by endogenous TSH.

Colloid goitre

A diffuse enlargement of the thyroid during adolescence is not unusual. This may be due to autoimmune thyroid disease which should be excluded. When thyroid function tests are normal and no antibodies are found, the diagnosis is usually of a colloid goitre. The thyroid enlargement usually resolves spontaneously, although it may be so great as to require surgery for cosmetic reasons.

Subacute thyroiditis

This term describes a thyroid gland acutely inflamed due to a variety of viral agents. It is self-limiting but may be very painful. Thyroid hormones 'leak' into the circulation and may give very bizarre biochemical results. Symptoms of hyperthyroidism may develop.

Treatment is with analgesics, non-steroidal antiinflammatory drugs and possibly corticosteroids. Propranolol may help symptoms of hyperthyroidism.

5

The adrenal gland

Clinical physiology

The fetal adrenal cortex becomes active during the second trimester and, at birth, it occupies 80% of the enlarged adrenal gland. The adult or definitive zones are scattered in groups around the periphery of the gland, and the adult configuration of three zones evolves with time, the zona reticularis not differentiating until middle childhood. It seems likely that cells gradually progress towards the centre of the adult adrenal cortex changing their function as they go. The enzymes of the adrenocortical cells are contained variously in microsomes and mitochondria so steroidogenesis requires coordination of mitochondrial and microsomal enzyme systems.

The outer zone of the adult cortex, the zona glomerulosa, comprises 10% of the cortical thickness. Its cells produce aldosterone and are under the control of the renin–angiotensin system which regulates both cholesterol uptake by the adrenal gland and also 18 hydroxylation of corticosterone (Fig. 5.1). This enzyme is not present elsewhere in the adrenal gland. The zona glomerulosa cells do not catalyse 17α-hydroxylation of progesterone, which is the principal substrate for the synthesis of the glucocorticoid and androgenic adrenal steroids.

Renin is synthesized by the juxtaglomerular apparatus and stored as a proenzyme in cells of the macula densa. When pulse pressure falls, plasma sodium concentration falls or plasma potassium concentration rises, this proteolytic enzyme hydrolyses angiotensin I from renin substrate (angiotensinogen), which is synthesized in the liver. Angiotensin converting enzyme, which is widely distributed in the vascular tissues and lung, converts angiotensin 1 to angiotensin II which has a very short half-life, being rapidly destroyed by angiotensinase. Angiotensin II stimulates the

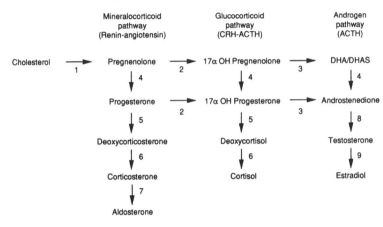

Enzymes
1. P450 cholesterol side chain cleavage
2. P450 17α-hydroxylase
3. 17,20-lyase (from same gene as 2)
4. 3β-hydroxysteroid dehydrogenase
5. 21-hydroxylase
6. 11β-hydroxylase
7. Aldosterone synthetase
8. 17β-hydroxysteroid dehydrogenase
9. Aromatase

Fig. 5.1. Pathways of adrenal steroid synthesis.

conversion of cholesterol to pregnenolone and the rate of conversion of corticosterone to aldosterone. The role of aldosterone is the fine-tuning of sodium and potassium exchange mainly in the renal distal tubule but also in the gut and sweat glands.

CRH–ACTH drive can increase cholesterol uptake by the adrenal gland to such an extent that aldosterone production is increased by mass action but this is an exceptional situation.

The zona fasciculata accounts for 75% of the volume of the cortex. It secretes primarily cortisol under the control of hypothalamic cortico-trophin releasing hormone(CRH) and pituitary adrenocorticotophic hormone (ACTH) but other steroid hormones may be produced, such as deoxycorticosterone and androstenedione, which may assume clinical importance if the ACTH drive to the zona fasciculata is increased.

ACTH is cleaved from a large precursor molecule, proopiomelano-cortin, which also contains the amino acid sequences of α-melanocyte-stimulating hormone (MSH), α-lipotrophin, β-endorphin, metenkephalin and β-MSH, the last two being found only within the central nervous system. ACTH causes an acute increase in the uptake of cholesterol by the

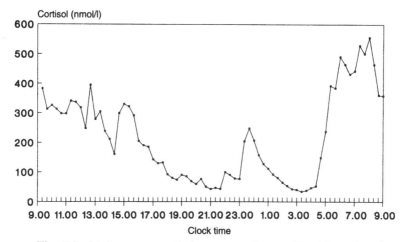

Fig. 5.2. 24 h serum cortisol concentration profile. Note that the concentration varies considerably around 0800 and 2400 h so that spot sample concentrations can give a misleading impression about diurnal variation.

adrenal gland. Chronic administration increases the cytochrome P-450 dependent enzymes (1,2,5 and 6 in Fig. 5.1).

The innermost zone, the zona reticularis, differentiates during middle childhood. It consists of cords of cells with interdigitating capillaries and secretes adrenal androgens, specifically dehydroepiandrosterone sulphate (DHAS). The control of steroid production in this zone is largely by ACTH but the part played by other hormones is not known.

Normal steroid values

Cortisol, cortisone and aldosterone are transported in serum bound to cortisol binding globulin (CBG) and albumin. Cortisol and cortisone are interconverted by the oxidoreductase 11β-hydroxysteroid dehydrogenase. In the adult the ratio of cortisol (active) to cortisone (inactive) is 5:1, but in fetal life it is 0.3:1. The liver is particularly active in reducing cortisone to cortisol; adipose tissue oxidizes cortisol to cortisone. The synthetic steroids, dexamethasone and 9α-fluorocortisol, are only weakly bound to CBG. Under ordinary circumstances, very little free cortisol is found in the plasma but, when total plasma cortisol concentration exceeds 600 nmol/l, the binding sites on CBG become saturated and plasma free cortisol and its urinary excretion rises.

ACTH and cortisol concentrations fluctuate continuously. The circadian rhythm emerges at about 6 months of age, and peak levels are generally higher in the morning than in the middle of the night. However, spot concentrations can be very misleading (See Fig. 5.2). 17α-hydroxy progesterone concentrations also have a diurnal rhythm; they are generally low in children but may rise under conditions of stress when ACTH levels are elevated.

Aldosterone circadian rhythm mirrors that of cortisol but concentrations are also markedly affected by changes of posture, which makes spot concentrations hard to interpret. In general, greater help is gained by comparing aldosterone concentrations with plasma renin activity and cortisol and 17α-hydroxyprogesterone levels with ACTH concentration than by measuring single samples.

Because of the rapid changes in plasma concentration, urinary steroid assays are particularly useful in paediatric practice. Complete urine collections are, however, very difficult to obtain from children. Some workers choose to express steroid excretion in terms of creatinine excretion thinking that the latter is constant; unfortunately, its excretion also varies from day to day, even if plasma levels do not change. In general, therefore, urine collections are useful to detect abnormal steroids or to determine ratios of excreted steroids rather than absolute amounts.

Thus, for example, the condition of 5α-reductase deficiency can be diagnosed more easily by comparing the ratio of 5β- to 5α-reduced metabolites of cortisol in urine than by comparing testosterone to dihydrotestosterone concentrations in blood samples after HCG stimulation. Congenital adrenal hyperplasia can be diagnosed in the newborn period not only by recognizing abnormal steroids but also by comparing ratios of excreted steroid metabolites to determine the nature of the enzymic block. This can be particularly helpful in salt losing states, since plasma assays for aldosterone, and particularly for its precursors, are not readily available.

Adrenal steroid deficiency

When the adrenal gland fails to function, there is potential for any combination of a salt-losing state, hypoglycemia and a lack of androgen secretion. Such a state may be acute or chronic and may arise through a defect in the adrenal gland itself or in the control mechanisms. The causes are shown in Table 5.1.

Table 5.1. *Causes of adrenal insufficiency*

Primary adrenal insufficiency
All zones
– Congenital adrenal hypoplasia
– Defects of adrenal steroid biosynthesis
– Adrenal hemorrhage
– Autoimmune adrenalitis
– Multiple endocrinopathy
– Infections (including effects of DIC)
– Adrenoleukodystrophy
– Iatrogenic, chemical or surgical
Zona glomerulosa (mineralocorticoids)
– Hypoaldosteronism
– Pseudohypoaldosteronism
Zona fasciculata
– Isolated glucocorticoid deficiency
– Congenital adrenal hyperplasia
– Iatrogenic
Zona reticularis
– 17,20 lyase deficiency
Secondary adrenal (ACTH) insufficiency
Congenital hypopituitarism
– multiple hormone deficiencies
– isolated ACTH deficiency
Tumours of the hypothalamo-pituitary axis
e.g. craniopharyngioma
Iatrogenic
e.g. surgery, radiotherapy, glucocorticoid therapy

Primary adrenal insufficiency

The commonest cause of adrenal insufficiency in the newborn is adrenal hemorrhage but the commonest cause in childhood is autoimmune disease. Recent data suggest that the autoantigen may be one of the key enzymes in steroid biosynthesis (17α-hydroxylase). If this is confirmed, it has important implications for the causation of other autoimmune disorders. Children with later onset of adrenal failure from this cause may present with hypoglycemia or with unexplained anorexia, vomiting and fatigue. Disorders of water balance may be complex, particularly if the cortisol deficiency is secondary to pituitary disease and ADH insufficiency is part of the symptom complex. Hyponatremia may, for example, be due to the inability to excrete a water load and have nothing to do with a coexisting mineralocorticoid problem. In this situation, the serum potassium concentration is important because it is always elevated when hyponatremia is due to aldosterone deficiency.

The key to making the diagnosis is not to forget its possibility in a chronically unwell child. Clinical examination for increased skin pigmentation will strongly point the diagnosis. It should always be suspected in families with autoimmune disease and in any patient who has autoimmune thyroid disease or diabetes mellitus. Presentation with addisonian symptoms generally precedes the dementia of adrenoleukodystrophy, and the measurement of very long chain fatty acids concentrations may be needed to make this (familial) diagnosis.

In infants, hypoglycemic episodes and/or a salt losing crisis are the predominant symptoms. Less serious degrees of cortisol deficiency may present with conjugated hyperbilirubinemia. Congenital adrenal hypoplasia may be sporadic or familial. The gland may be small or absent (anencephalic pattern), hypoplastic but with three normally differentiated zones (miniature pattern) or its architecture may be disordered with large abnormal cells (cytomegalic pattern). The cytomegalic pattern is inherited in an X-linked fashion, the miniature pattern as an autosomal recessive and all three patterns occur sporadically.

A warning that this condition may be present can be derived from the absence of maternal estriol excretion during pregnancy in the presence of an apparently healthy fetus. When the child is born, it rapidly exhibits severe symptoms of profound salt loss and hypoglycemia, as do all children with acute adrenal failure. These include vomiting (due to glucocorticoid deficiency), pallor and shock (due to mineralocorticoid deficiency).

Deficiencies of the enzyme systems incorporating cholesterol into the adrenal gland and deficiency of 3β-hydroxysteroid dehydrogenase will present similarly in the newborn period (see section on congenital adrenal hyperplasia, page 109), as will the other causes of primary adrenal insufficiency later in childhood, although a more insidious presentation with intermittent symptoms can cause much clinical confusion.

Isolated deficiencies of adrenal steroid hormones present as salt losing states (see Chapter 6) or with hypoglycemia. Since any ill baby may become hypoglycemic, this finding cannot be assumed to be due to glucocorticoid deficiency without biochemical confirmation. Isolated glucocorticoid deficiency is rare and may be only the initial presentation of a progressive adrenal failure. I have seen one child take 15 years to develop a salt wasting tendency having presented with episodic hypoglycemia due to glucocorticoid deficiency, which was relieved by steroid medication. Over the years plasma renin activity was repeatedly found to be normal and the patient also responded normally to the challenge of a low salt diet. When isolated glucocorticoid deficiency is associated with achalasia and alachryma, a condition which runs in families, it probably does not progress to a complete addisonian picture.

The abnormalities confined to the individual zones will present with the relevant symptoms. The hallmark to distinguish pseudohypoaldosteronism from the real deficiency is the failure to respond to mineralocorticoid replacement therapy (see Chapter 6, page 121). Adrenal androgen deficiency is a disorder primarily affecting females if testicular function is retained; this will not, of course, be the case in 17,20 lyase deficiency.

Secondary adrenal insufficiency

This must be suspected whenever a child presents with hypopituitarism. GH insufficiency is much the most common of such presentations, and gonadotrophin insufficiency comes not far behind in terms of prevalence. Isolated ACTH deficiency is very rare but ACTH deficiency combined with other pituitary hormone problems is not uncommon, especially when the hypopituitary state is congenital or the result of the presence or the treatment of an intracranial neoplasm. ACTH deficiency is not an uncommon sequela of cranial irradiation but it may not declare itself for many years, certainly not until long after GH deficiency has been diagnosed, and possibly not until after the treatment for this has been completed. In congenital hypopituitarism, there may be obvious midline abnormalities, but the infant may present simply with hypoglycemia and unexplained jaundice (due to conjugated hyperbilirubinemia) and only later show signs of hypothyroidism and growth failure secondary to GH deficiency. LH deficiency may present with micropenis.

Hyporeninemic hypoaldosteronism is well recognized in adult patients with chronic renal disease usually associated with diabetes mellitus but it is very rare in children. A pair of siblings with a partially affected father has been described from France in whom hypoaldosteronism was attributed to congenital deficiency of renin activity and/or angiotensinogen production.

Management

Once the diagnosis has been suspected, either clinically or from preliminary biochemical results (hyponatremia and hyperkalemia), the diagnosis is easy to confirm. A measurement of serum cortisol concentration should be made and parallelled with a measurement of serum ACTH concentration. (The latter specimen needs to be separated in a cool centrifuge and frozen without delay.) Blood should also be obtained for the estimation of plasma aldosterone concentration and renin activity. (The latter specimen needs to be collected in EDTA).

If the serum cortisol concentration is low or normal and the ACTH raised, the diagnosis of primary glucocorticoid deficiency is confirmed. A similar discrepancy between aldosterone and renin concentrations confirms a diagnosis of primary mineralocorticoid deficiency.

If the serum cortisol concentration is low and the ACTH concentration is also low, secondary glucocorticoid deficiency may be diagnosed: this leads to investigation of the rest of the hypothalamo-pituitary axis and to (MR) imaging of that area.

If there is reason to believe that secondary hypoadrenalism is likely, such as after surgery and/or radiotherapy for a craniopharyngioma, and the basal cortisol concentration is normal, it may be necessary to test the ability of the hypothalamo-pituitary–adrenal axis to respond to stress. This can be achieved by injecting glucagon, by lowering blood glucose through the injection of insulin or by administering metyrapone (although I do not advise this test). It can also be inferred by the administration of a low dose (500 ng/m^2) of ACTH. These tests are discussed further in chapter 10 (page 163).

Hyporeninemic hypoaldosteronism would be diagnosed by the finding of low levels of plasma renin activity and aldosterone in a patient with hyponatremia and hyperkalemia.

Treatment

Addisonian crisis means what it says, and urgent measures are needed to restore plasma volume and cardiac output. When in doubt, it is better to introduce steroid replacement medications and to revisit the diagnosis later once the emergency has passed.

In the acute situation, nobody would try to use a glucocorticoid other than cortisol (hydrocortisone) which is what the child lacks. The cortisol secretion rate in childhood is as fixed as any biological parameter can be at 12.5 mg/m^2/24 h, and subsequent replacement should be based on this figure after making allowance for taking the medication enterally. A safe oral replacement dose of hydrocortisone is 15 mg/m^2/24 h, and this should be given in a twice daily regimen, two-thirds of the dose in the morning and one-third at night. There is no place in my opinion for the administration of cortisone acetate in 1992. A very few children may need a longer acting steroid at night to prevent nocturnal hypoglycemia and, in them, but only in them, I sometimes use prednisolone at night. This does sometimes cause growth suppression but the need for it does not usually last very long.

Hydrocortisone does have some mineralocorticoid activity but it is a bad mistake to try to use it to control a salt-losing state due to mineralocorticoid deficiency. Replacement for this is needed with 9α-fluorocortisol (fludro-cortisone acetate, trade name Florinef) in a dose of $150\ \mu g/m^2/24$ h, which is given as a single morning dose. As fludrocortisone has the same glucocorticoid activity as dexamethasone, it helps with the glucocorticoid medication and, in a child with nocturnal symptoms of hypocortisolemia, the administration of all or part of the dose of fludrocortisone in the evening may be helpful because of its duration of action.

The adequacy of replacement may be checked clinically by ensuring an absence of symptoms, by growth assessment and biochemically by measuring concentrations of cortisol, ACTH and plasma renin activity. Over the years, however, I have had so little trouble by carefully titrating the doses of replacement medication to size (being particularly careful during puberty) that I am inclined to seek other causes, specifically lack of compliance, rather than pursue biochemical tests, which are undertaken in the rather artificial setting of a hospital day, to explain persisting or recurring symptoms.

Adrenal steroid excess

The commonest cause of steroid excess is iatrogenic but primary and secondary adrenocortical overactivity, although much less common, have important consequences and need special attention to diagnosis and management. The causes are shown in Table 5.2. Primary and secondary mineralocorticoid excess will be discussed in Chapter 6.

Primary adrenal disorders

Cushing syndrome is the term traditionally applied to glucocorticoid excess whether that be due to hypersecretion of steroids or iatrogenic. In children with adrenal disorders, Cushing disease, adrenal steroid excess secondary to ACTH drive (see below), is overwhelmingly the commonest cause and this affects the production (and results in the consequences) of steroids from all three cortical zones, so I think that the imprecision of the term Cushing syndrome does not serve well.

Table 5.2. *Causes of adrenal steroid excess*

Primary adrenal disorders
  Glucocorticoid excess
    Nodular adrenal hyperplasia
    Adrenal neoplasm
  Mineralocorticoid excess
    Adrenal neoplasm (Conn syndrome)
    Dexamethasone-suppressible hyperaldosteronism
    CAH (11β and 17α-hydroxylase)
  Androgen excess
    Adrenal neoplasm
    CAH (11β and 21-hydroxylase)
    Late onset CAH
    'Premature adrenarche'
Secondary adrenal hyperplasia
  CRH and ACTH secreting tumours
  Renin secreting tumours
  Bartter syndrome
Iatrogenic

CAH = Congenital adrenal hyperplasia.

In the rare instances in children when glucocorticoids are secreted in excess alone by the adrenal cortex, bilateral nodular adrenal hyperplasia may be responsible but adrenal neoplasm, benign or malignant, is more frequent. In my experience, however, adrenal carcinoma much more frequently presents with evidence of marked androgen excess (pubic hair, acne, hirsutism and cliteromegaly, because the incidence is higher in girls) than with Cushing syndrome.

The clinical features of Cushing syndrome are well known (obesity, hypertension and signs of moderate androgen excess) but the effect on growth varies according to the relative amounts of steroids excreted, which depends on age. In a young child, obesity and growth arrest are characteristic; in an older child, the secretion of adrenal androgens may actually stimulate growth and mislead the clinician. The cause of the obesity is (as always) hard to define, but it certainly follows a period of increased calorie intake at a time when growth is suppressed probably due to abnormalities distal to the generation of IGF-I. This does not explain the curious central distribution of fat deposition which is so characteristic. Capillary fragility and dermal thinning so common in adult patients are rare in children. The presentation is usually with symptoms of hypertension, obesity, androgen excess or growth arrest.

The various forms of congenital adrenal hyperplasia (see below) present with mineralocorticoid and androgen excess: by definition, cortisol secretion is impaired. 'Premature adrenarche' has been discussed previously (Chapter 3 on page 61).

Secondary adrenal hyperplasia

Cushing syndrome in children not due to administered steroids is nearly always due to a disorder of feedback of cortisol on CRH–ACTH secretion which leads to a pituitary adenoma. The distinction between primary and secondary adrenal disease in adult patients with Cushing syndrome can be extremely difficult, which explains the plethora of tests employed, none of which is completely reliable. In children, the results of the tests may be equally confusing but the remedy is nearly always in pituitary surgery. Ectopic production of CRH or ACTH is extremely unusual in children.

Iatrogenic Cushing syndrome is the commonest and purest form of the disorder. It results in obesity and also in hypertension even if pure glucocorticoids are administered. The growth suppression secondary to steroid medication remains something of a mystery. It cannot all be attributed to abnormal GH secretion and does not seem to be attributable to a failure of IGF generation. There seems to be a failure of translation of the IGF message, which probably explains why the administration of GH to children made short by steroid medication is such a dismal exercise. What is certainly true and cannot be overemphasized is that the disorders for which steroids are prescribed and in which they are life-saving are much more serious than short stature. The control of disease must come first, and concern about the side effects second; this applies particularly to asthma where growth delay usually deals with the problem of short stature in the end.

Management

When a child is suspected of having steroid excess, the first step is to confirm that this is the case, which may be easier said than done. As indicated previously, the excretion of urinary free cortisol will not rise until cortisol binding in serum is exceeded and the symptoms of steroid excess may well precede this. It is always said that the hallmark of Cushing syndrome is the loss of diurnal variation and this is certainly true. However, as Fig. 5.2 showed, there is often a rise of cortisol concentration around midnight in normal subjects and so if only two samples are taken at 2400 h and 0800 h and they happen to coincide with a peak and trough at those times, a false diagnosis will be made.

The most reliable diagnoses are made by relating measurements of urinary steroid excretion of cortisol and androgen metabolites using group analyses, which are now rarely available, or gas–liquid chromatography to body surface area. A complementary method is to examine a profile of serum cortisol concentration, the longer the better but for not less than two hours at 20 minute intervals in the middle of the night and in the early morning. The concentrations achieved at these times should be compared with a few concentrations of ACTH.

Where cortisol concentrations are high and ACTH is detectable, Cushing disease may be diagnosed with confidence. The next step is high resolution (MR) imaging of the pituitary prior to transsphenoidal exploration of the pituitary fossa. We have found that trying to localize an adenoma by its hormonal excretion and response to stimuli is very unrewarding in children so, if the diagnosis is sure and even if the imaging does not clearly reveal the source of the problem, we would proceed to pituitary exploration and trust the surgeon to find and remove the adenoma. This counsel may be biased by the skill of the neurosurgeon with whom I work but it has served our patients well.

It is important not to be disappointed by the histological examination of the specimen removed: it is nearly always reported as normal pituitary tissue but what matters is whether the condition of the patient remits and whether any concomitant pituitary hormone deficiency has resulted from the intervention. In selective adenomectomy this is rare and postoperative diabetes insipidus is nearly always transient. Where the condition has not remitted or recurs, which is not uncommon because the feedback disorder has not been eliminated by surgery, reoperation is the next step leading, ultimately, to total hypophysectomy which necessitates replacement therapy with thyroxine, hydrocortisone, gonadotrophins or sex steroids, as well as GH and DDAVP (see Chapter 9). Using this strategy, we have not had to resort to adrenalectomy (with its danger of Nelson syndrome, unrestrained ACTH and MSH secretion from the pituitary tumour), pituitary irradiation or medical management with metyrapone or amino-glutethimide. Whether adrenalectomy and regular MR imaging to detect the pituitary tumour of Nelson syndrome is a good idea I do not know. What I do know is that treating a Nelson tumour is more difficult than pituitary hormone replacement, so I prefer to advise hypophysectomy.

Where cortisol is high and ACTH low, it is necessary to proceed to adrenal imaging. Ultrasonography, which is easy for the patient, is not a good medium to choose for this purpose. The most skilled operators find adrenal ultrasound very difficult to interpret and CT is greatly to be preferred. MR imaging is probably less good in this area. The use of iodocholesterol scintigraphy and venous catheterization of the adrenal veins is rare now because of improvements in other imaging methodologies. Where an adrenal tumour is defined, it should be removed surgically.

Where cortisol is high and ACTH very high, a search has to be instituted to find the source of the ectopic hormone production. A lung carcinoid is probably first on the list in children and CT scanning of the lungs the best way to identify it. Venous catheterization and stimulation with CRH may be needed to localize an ectopic source of ACTH.

If androgen excess is the primary presenting feature of steroid excess, the probable cause is an adrenal adenoma or carcinoma. The latter may be familial and associated with osteosarcoma. Gas–liquid chromatographic separation of urinary steroid metabolites and indentification of steroids by mass spectroscopy is the best method of diagnosis and the findings can have prognostic value. The tumours should be identifiable by CT, and possibly by selective venous catheterization, and should be removed. Histological examination may be unable to determine whether a tumour is benign or malignant. If it has been removed completely, even if there has been some local invasion of the adrenal capsule or of the adrenal vein, there is no place for preventive chemotherapy, and radiotherapy does not have a role. Regular clinical follow-up to detect a recurrence of symptoms and urinary steroid analysis is required; should the patient relapse, it is likely to be with distant metastases, and chemotherapy is the only (and forlorn) hope.

Congenital adrenal hyperplasia

When there is an enzymic block in the synthesis of cortisol, CRH–ACTH drive to the adrenal gland promotes the incorporation of cholesterol into the adrenal cortex (the hyperplasia seen macroscopically which gave the condition its name). The effects of the condition depend first upon which of the adrenal steroids the cortex is unable to synthesize and second upon the steroids which are secreted in excess as a result of the ACTH drive and the accumulation of the substrate steroid which precedes the block. The varieties of CAH and their effects are shown in Table 5.3, which should be read in the context of the pathways of adrenal steroid biosynthesis (Fig. 5.1).

Table 5.3. *Varieties of congenital adrenal hyperplasia and their effects*

| Enzyme defect | Ambiguous genitalia in genotypic | | Salt loss | Hyper-tension | Puberty |
	Males	Females			
Cholesterol side chain cleavage	+	–	+	–	Absent
3β-hydroxysteroid dehydrogenase	+	+	+	–	Absent
17α-hydroxylase	+	–	–	+	Absent
21-hydroxylase	–	+	+	–	Precocious
11β-hydroxylase	–	+	–	+	Precocious

CAH may present with:

- ambiguity of the genitalia
- a salt losing crisis in the newborn period
- hypertension
- precocious puberty in males
- signs of androgen excess in females
- 'bilateral cryptorchidism' and breast development in puberty, i.e. females raised inappropriately as males.

These are all indications to think of the diagnosis which may be confirmed by demonstrating:

1. a low or normal cortisol concentration in the presence of elevated ACTH concentrations,
2. the presence of precursor steroids in blood in abnormal concentrations (e.g. 17α-hydroxyprogesterone),
3. the identification of urinary steroid metabolites in abnormally high or low quantities which will enable the enzymic block to be defined.

Ambiguous genitalia

If testosterone cannot be synthesized in sufficient quantity, male sexual differentiation will be inadequate. In cholesterol side chain cleavage(SCC) deficiency, there may be completely normal external female genitalia in a male baby and such a patient has to be reared as a female, even though there is no uterus present.

In 3β-hydroxysteroid dehydrogenase (HSD) deficiency, the DHA secreted will be inadequate fully to masculinize a male baby but sufficient to masculinize the external genitalia of a female fetus. The former need some additional testosterone (Sustanon 25 mg IM at monthly intervals until the phallus is of normal size, which usually takes three injections) and the latter clitoral reduction.

The degree of enzymic block in 17α hydroxylase deficiency is usually sufficient to prevent masculinization of a male fetus and such patients present later as females with hypertension who are found to have no uterus present. Female sexual differentiation is, of course, normal: a uterus is present but puberty has to be induced.

With deficiencies at 21- or 11β hydroxylase, males are unaffected but female infants will be masculinized as a result of exposure to DHA, androstenedione and testosterone *in utero* and will require corrective surgery (see Chapter 1).

Water balance

Where aldosterone biosynthesis is impaired (cholesterol-SCC, 3β HSD and 21 hydroxylase deficiencies), a salt losing crisis may be expected within the first 10 days of birth. The first sign of this is a rising serum potassium concentration; should this occur, samples should be taken for estimation of plasma renin activity and aldosterone concentration (as well as the samples needed for the confirmation of the diagnosis – see above) and the baby should be started on salt supplements and mineralocorticoid replacement *before* the serum sodium concentration starts to fall. In this way a hypotensive crisis can be averted and necrotizing enterocolitis (commonly seen in CAH) and pituitary infarction (less commonly seen but very important) prevented. Trying to forecast a salt-losing crisis by determining urinary sodium loss is not useful, because the sodium intake is difficult to assess, because the absolute urinary sodium loss is not very great but greater than the neonate (who is in a precarious salt balance anyway) can stand and because the loss is also in the faeces and sweat and therefore difficult to measure. Whether all patients with 21 hydroxylase deficiency harbour a salt losing tendency is much debated; for practical purposes, it seems to be more or less invariable that a serious degree of genital ambiguity is associated with salt loss but female patients do present later in life with virilization without salt loss and so may males with signs of androgen excess in childhood or infertility later.

Where mineralocorticoid synthesis can proceed normally, the ACTH drive caused by cortisol deficiency results in hypertension. In 17α-hydroxylase deficiency, this is because of hyperaldosteronism. The adrenal zones function relatively independently; thus there are different 11β-hydroxylase systems in the zonae fasciculata and glomerulosa. If the 11β-hydroxyiase system is deficint only in the zona fasciculata, the female patient with CAH will have ambiguous genitalia and the male exhibit precocious puberty. The blood pressure will be unaffected. If, however, the same enzymic deficiency affects the mineralocorticoid pathway, the precursor steroid (desoxycorticosterone) has sufficient mineralocorticoid activity to cause very severe (malignant) hypertension. This can be cured by suppressing ACTH drive using cortisol, but the enzymic block in the mineralocorticoid pathway may be sufficiently dense for a salt losing tendency to become unmasked in the treated patient unstimulated by ACTH. Paradoxically, such patients may therefore require both gluco-corticoid and mineralocorticoid replacement, the latter to suppress the renin–angiotensin drive of the (now salt-losing) zona glomerulosa.

Hypertension is rarely a problem in the early years of life, although it can be severe (and even malignant and lethal) before the age of 5 years. Hypoglycemia, the prime symptom of glucocorticoid deficiency, is not usually a problem for the patient with CAH because CRH–ACTH drive is usually sufficient to maintain a normal cortisol production rate in the basal state. If the patient becomes stressed by salt loss and cortisol production would then be expected to rise, it cannot do so because it is already maximal. Hypoglycemia may then become a serious and life-threatening problem which requires attention.

Puberty

If the level of the enzymic deficiency prevents sex steroid synthesis, puberty obviously cannot occur, and the patient requires sex steroid replacement.

If CRH–ACTH drive can promote testosterone synthesis (in 21- and 11β-hydroxylase deficiencies), males will enter puberty precociously, and females will become masculinized.

For reasons not yet clear, all females with CAH (at least those with 21-hydroxylase deficiency which is much the commonest form of CAH) develop polycystic ovaries (PCO). Acne, hirsutism, delayed menarche, and irregular scanty periods, are all characteristics of the PCO syndrome (together with obesity). It is not clear whether the gene for PCO colocates with that for 21-hydroxylase, whether PCO is predetermined by fetal exposure to androgens, or whether the androgenic excess seen inter-mittently in females treated for CAH causes a polycystic change.

Fertility used to be regarded as exceptional in male patients with CAH. This was probably because they were undertreated and the testosterone from their adrenal glands suppressed the hypothalamo-pituitary–testicular axis. Certainly, when male adolescents default on treatment, the result can be seen in the measurement of their testicular volume. Since this can be restored to normal by treatment, the prognosis for reproductive capability is good.

Unfortunately, the same cannot be said for females. As well as the anatomical and psychological problems caused by genital ambiguity and its surgical correction, females face the additional problems of PCOS. Pregnancy is certainly possible and frequently recorded in the adequately replaced female with CAH but there is a high incidence of delay in conceiving and early pregnancy loss of the baby. Once the first trimester has passed, things proceed quite normally.

Management

Whenever the diagnosis of CAH is suspected, specimens of blood and urine are required to define the nature of the enzymic deficiency. Although 21 hydroxylase deficiency is the commonest of the varieties, the different consequences of failing to diagnose the other varieties are considerable. A definitive diagnosis of the enzyme block should be reached.

Pelvic ultrasound with or without radiographic contrast examination should define the extent of gynaecological or urological problem and the appropriate specialist should be enrolled to deal with it certainly within the first 12 and possibly first 3 months of life.

Once blood and urine specimens have been gathered, and especially if the patient is a baby and is in any way unwell, therapy should be commenced. As indicated, we would not hesitate to treat a rising potassium concentration with mineralocorticoid replacement and salt supplements.

Mineralocorticoid replacement is given in the form of *tablets* of 9α-fluorocortisol (fludrocortisone, trade name Florinef) in a dose of 150 μg/m^2/24 h to be taken orally daily. *There is no method of reliably suspending this medication* and pharmacists must be told specifically not to attempt to do so. The administration of crushed parts of tablets is not a problem for parents, but I have seen countless instances of babies becoming sick through a failure to take the active ingredient of a suspension.

Mineralocorticoid replacement has an effect only if salt intake is sufficient. Administration of huge doses of fludrocortisone to a normal volunteer on a low salt diet simply results in a potassium diuresis. All salt-losing patients, particularly those recovering from a period of unrestrained salt loss (such as newborn infants, especially if they are breast fed), need salt supplements. The amount can vary from double the normal daily requirement (2 mmol/kg/24 h) to several times that level. Initial salt supplements should err on the generous side to replace previous losses and the patient should be stabilized on mineralocorticoid replacement and salt supplements tailored to generate a normal sodium concentration.

When the patient starts to take (unmodified) cow's milk, salt supplements can be omitted in a temperate climate but, where the ambient temperature rises to the higher 20 °C, and always when it is in excess of 30 °C, patients are safer and more comfortable and their condition is better controlled with a salt supplement of 1–2 mmol/kg/24 h.

Mineralocorticoid therapy should be scrupulously tailored to body surface area. I have yet to see or hear of a patient in whom the dose recommended fails to keep the plasma renin activity normal so if it is raised on a routine check, the dose, the medication, the form in which it is administered or a lack of compliance must be presumed in the first instance.

Mineralocorticoid replacement is more important for the safety and well-being of the patient with CAH than glucocorticoid replacement and yet the latter attracts much more attention, even though hypoglycemia is not a common problem in the clinical management of these patients – at least not in my experience, but I do stress the dangers of omitting mineralocorticoid replacement to my patients and fludrocortisone has a useful glucocorticoid action.

To suppress CRH–ACTH drive of unwanted steroids, and to replace cortisol secretion, patients need hydrocortisone replacement in a dose of 15–25 mg/m²/24 h. No other glucocorticoid medication is acceptable, except in exceptional circumstances (see below). The tolerance to variations in dosage of glucocorticoid is much greater than for mineralocorticoids; as long as the replacement dose of mineralocorticoid is adequate and plasma renin activity has been checked on at least one occasion to confirm that it is appropriate for that particular patient, glucocorticoid replacement is not as critical as some workers have claimed. Glucocorticoid medication needs increasing in times of serious stress but not for every trivial illness if other medications are adequate. Still, it is better to err on the side of safety than conservatism.

For the monitoring of glucocorticoid replacement, some physicians like to measure profiles or spot concentrations of steroid hormones in blood, saliva or urine. For patients with 21-hydroxylase deficiency, the steroid most usually pursued is 17-hydroxyprogesterone or its urinary metabolite pregnanetriol. The problem is that any measurement is only as good as the period over which it is taken; 17-hydroxyprogesterone has a diurnal variation and is subject to stress. Biochemical measurement cannot detect non-compliance in this condition (cf. hypothyroidism); it can only assess the adequacy of a given dose. I am unconvinced that the pursuit of biochemical purity in terms of glucocorticoid replacement benefits the patient.

Children exposed to testosterone grow fast and advance their bone age excessively quickly. Children exposed to excessive glucocorticoids grow slowly and advance their bone age more slowly than normal but not as slowly as they grow. Thus growth assessment provides the perfect method for ensuring adequacy and appropriateness of glucocorticoid medication.

My practice is to take time and trouble to define the diagnosis. Patients are then adequately replaced with mineralocorticoid and this is checked by measuring plasma renin activity. The patient is started on hydrocortisone replacement and growth is monitored initially every 3–4 months, routinely every 6 months and more frequently at times of rapid change in surface area (early infancy and puberty). If all is well, no regular blood tests are performed. Blood pressure should be monitored and plasma renin activity checked every year or so.

If things do not go as expected, a number of snags may be responsible. Compliance is the first. Next, is an error in prescribing. Next, is another condition which may or may not be associated with CAH. As indicated, GH insufficiency is a strong candidate if the initial illness was a severe one with hypotensive crises. In cases of doubt, I do not hesitate to readmit the patient to hospital and go over the whole of the diagnostic and dose finding schedule again, but I rarely have to resort to this and my patients very rarely darken the doors of the in-patient unit from the time of diagnosis till their transfer to the adult endocrine unit, except for gynaecological and urological treatments.

Genetic aspects

The molecular genetic basis of 21-hydroxylase deficiency has been studied thoroughly and the results have considerable practical value. The molecular genetic basis of the other (much less common) forms of CAH is not well established.

The gene encoding the microsomal cytochrome P450 21-hydroxylase enzyme system (CYP21 or CYP21B) and a pseudogene (CYP21P or

CYP21A) are located in the HLA complex about 30 kilobases apart adjacent to, and alternating with, C4B and C4A genes encoding the fourth component of serum complement. All mutations causing 21-hydroxylase deficiency appear to result from recombinations between CYP21B and CYP21A resulting either in deletion of the former or transfer to CYP21B of deleterious mutations normally present in the CYP21A pseudogene.

Particular mutations and the degree of enzymatic compromise caused by each may be correlated with the different forms of 21 hydroxylase deficiency but obviously the genes on both chromosomes have to be affected or there has to be a deletion of the other CYP21B locus for any variety of the disease to be manifest. Point (single amino acid) deletions lead to up to 50% diminution in 21-hydroxylase activity which is associated with relatively minor symptoms of virilization which might occur in heterozygote parents of an affected child (non-classical or late-onset disease).

Deletions of longer sequences may result in up to 99% loss of function this manifests with severe virilization but mineralocorticoid secretion remains adequate because aldosterone is normally secreted at a rate 100–1000 times lower than that of cortisol, so that 21-hydroxylase activity has to be very low indeed before it becomes rate limiting in mineralo-corticoid synthesis. Such a patient presents with non-salt losing (simple virilizing) 21-hydroxylase deficiency. Complete deletion of the gene or more extensive base deletions result in complete loss of 21-hydroxylase deficiency: such a patient presents in the newborn period with classical severe salt-losing CAH.

Antenatal diagnosis and treatment

In a family to whom a child affected with CAH due to 21-hydroxylase has been born it may be possible to recognize in the child and in the parents the antecedent genetic explanations of the problem. If this is the case, it is possible to obtain a sample of fetal tissue from an unborn child and to forecast whether or not that child is affected in the same way as its sibling.

In times gone by, an antenatal diagnosis could be obtained from the measurement of the concentration of excreted steroids in the amniotic fluid (obtained at about 18 weeks of gestation by amniocentesis) or by the culture of fibroblasts and the determination of HLA status, which segregates with the CAH genes because of their colocation on chromosome 6. This was late in a pregnancy and the diagnosis took too long.

The modern technique is to obtain a chorionic villus sample, to extract fetal DNA from it, to amplify the relavent genetic sequence by the polymerase chain reaction and to seek the genetic defect which is known to exist in the previously affected sibling. This takes 48 hours and, if the genetic markers are present, this fetus is also affected with 21-hydroxylase deficiency.

The point of all this is to administer steroid medication to the fetus via the mother to suppress the hypothalamo-pituitary–adrenal axis to prevent the elaboration of androgens under CRH–ACTH drive and thereby reduce or eliminate genital ambiguity in an affected female fetus.

In practical terms what is done is this. The genetic basis of the disease in the proband is defined. As soon as the mother becomes pregnant again (and this is confirmed biochemically and/or ultrasonically by 6 weeks of gestation), she commences treatment with dexamethasone 0.25 mg tds. At 12 weeks or thereabout a chorion villus biopsy is performed and the DNA examined as above for CAH markers and also for Y chromosomal material. If the baby is not affected, the treatment is stopped. If the fetus is male and affected, the treatment is stopped but the newborn nursery should be alerted for the impending salt loss. If the fetus is female and affected, the treatment is continued to term.

The information gathered could, of course, be used as an indication to terminate a pregnancy of an affected child male or female, but few parents in my experience choose to use it in this way. Many see the taking of medication throughout pregnancy as a bigger hurdle than the disease itself and, in this situation, there is not much point in attempting an antenatal diagnosis. These are considerations which require much time and discussion; the techniques are not widely available and I advise physicians inexperienced in this field, and without access to the relevant techniques, to seek help from an experienced centre.

Non-classical (late onset) CAH

Point mutations of amino acids are relatively common in the 21 hydroxylase gene. In certain populations, such as the Jews of Eastern European (Ashkenazi) extraction, the gene frequency may be more than 10%. The mutation results in an enzyme that has about 50% of normal activity for the hydroxylation of 17α-hydroxyprogesterone. This may be sufficient in some patients to cause antenatal virilization but it may not present until adrenarche, puberty or even later in life with signs of androgen excess (acne, hirsutism, polycystic ovaries, etc). Treatment is, of course, to replace cortisol to prevent CRH–ACTH drive of unwanted steroids.

Adrenomedullary dysfunction

Adrenomedullary deficiency

Failure of the adrenal medulla is very uncommon. It causes hypotension and, more importantly, hypoglycemia but the hormones of the adrenal cortex are more important in this respect and children do not need adrenomedullary replacement treatment after adrenalectomy or adrenal destruction by hemorrhage. The condition of familial dysautonomia (Riley–Day syndrome), which is due to a hereditary deficiency of dopamine-β-hydroxylase, is, however, quite a different story. Here, there is a widespread disorder of function which includes dysphagia, instability of blood pressure, motor disability, lack of pain sensation and, most characteristically, a lack of tears. Treatment is supportive.

Adrenomedullary hyperfunction

Tumours secreting catecholamines cause hypertension and that subject will be covered in Chapter 6. Pheochromocytoma may be isolated or associated with multiple endocrine neoplasms (MEN II) or with various neurocutaneous syndromes such as multiple fibromatoses, Hippel–von Lindau disease, Sturge–Weber syndrome and tuberous sclerosis.

6

Salt and water balance

The magnitude of the glomerular filtrate requires very special mechanisms for the conservation of water and two of them, the exchange of sodium for potassium in the distal tubule under the control of renin and aldosterone and the control of free water excretion in the collecting duct by vasopressin (antidiuretic hormone, ADH), are under endocrine control.

Hyponatremia

All babies teeter on the brink of salt and water loss, because the osmolality of the renal medulla has not attained the level it needs for adequate reabsorption of water from the loop of Henle, even though a decreased glomerular perfusion protects the immature renal tubules. In early postnatal life, blood is distributed preferentially to the juxtamedullary area to nephrons with a higher capacity than the superficial ones to reabsorb sodium, but obligatory sodium reabsorption in the proximal tubule is limited so the neonate has a greater dependence on distal tubular function. Preterm infants are especially at risk of hyponatremia.

The renin–angiotensin system is functional in the fetus, and levels of renin activity, angiotensin and aldosterone are very high in the newborn. If these mechanisms are defective in any way, urinary sodium loss can rapidly cause serious salt depletion, even though the absolute loss of sodium may not be very great.

There is considerable clinical variability in the presentation of a salt-losing state ranging from moderate failure to thrive to a life-threatening salt-losing crisis. The serum sodium concentration alone may be misleading in such a situation. If the loss of water and sodium are equivalent, for example, the serum sodium concentration may be near normal even though there is serious salt depletion. Conversely, in an older patient, the inability to excrete a water load due to glucocorticoid insufficiency may give rise to apparent hyponatremia, even though total body sodium is increased. The key to establishing the real position is the measurement of plasma renin activity which will be elevated in the former situation and suppressed in the latter.

Salt loss in children may be gastrointestinal or urinary; in the case of urinary loss, the cause may be renal or adrenal. When there is renal disease (renal dysplasia, obstructive uropathy or renal tubular dysfunction) both sodium and potassium are lost so that the serum concentrations of both sodium and potassium are low. If necessary, the disorder can be proved to be of renal origin if the renin and aldosterone levels are both demonstrated to be high.

In the face of hyperkalemia, hyponatremia is likely to be due to adrenal disease, such as congenital adrenal hypoplasia, the salt losing varieties of congenital adrenal hyperplasia, Addison disease or defects in aldosterone biosynthesis or action. The first three conditions have been covered in Chapter 5.

Defects of aldosterone biosynthesis

Defects of aldosterone synthetase (18 oxidation or 18 hydroxylation – see Fig. 5.1) lead to an inability to synthesize aldosterone when the gluco-corticoid pathway is intact. Children present in infancy with a salt-losing crisis or failure to thrive. Hyponatremia and hyperkalemia rapidly point the diagnosis which is confirmed by measuring plasma renin activity and comparing its high level with a low concentration of aldosterone. GC–MS separation and identification of urinary steroid metabolites will define the level of the enzymic block. When mineralocorticoid and salt replacement has been instituted, the normality of the glucocorticoid pathway can be confirmed but it must be remembered that when the patient is ill concentrations of ACTH and cortisol precursors may well be (appropriately) elevated and this may cause diagnostic confusion.

The doses of salt and of 9α-fluorocortisol may need initially to be very high because of the competition for mineralocorticoid binding with aldosterone precursor steroids. They later resume the normal doses ($150 \mu g/m^2/24$ h for fludrocortisone and a variable salt supplement titrated against the serum sodium concentration) and will be required for life.

The syndrome of hyporeninemic hypoaldosteronism has been mentioned previously (page 104).

Pseudohypoaldosteronism

The hallmark of this condition, which presents in the same way as aldosterone deficiency, is the finding of an elevated concentration of plasma aldosterone. The nature of the defective action of aldosterone is not clear but, of course, mineralocorticoid replacement is ineffective.

These children have to be treated with large quantities of salt supplement. Indomethacin can be a useful addition to therapy by decreasing glomerular filtrate and improving proximal tubular sodium reabsorption.

Bartter syndrome

Hyperreninemic hyperaldosteronism presents with failure to thrive, vomiting, weakness and fatigue. It may just present with short stature. Biochemical findings must include hypokalemia, hypochloremia, alkalosis and normal blood pressure in the presence of hyperreninemia. There is a widespread disorder of renal function, the exact mechanism of which is not known.

Treatment is not very satisfactory with potassium and sodium supplementation. Potassium sparing diuretics may help, as may indomethacin and other inhibitors of prostaglandin synthesis. The prognosis is better with these measures because wide swings of sodium and potassium concentrations are avoided but poor growth and chronic renal failure remain problems in some patients.

Endocrine hypertension

Mild hypertension in children, which is probably essential hypertension, is important because of its longstanding contribution to atherosclerotic cardiovascular disease. The aetiology is much disputed but if treatment of mild hypertension is important for adults, as it seems to be, it must be more important for children who have to endure the condition for longer.

Severe hypertension needs urgent treatment to prevent cerebral haemorrhage, blindness and renal failure. It needs to be taken very seriously and too few children have their blood pressure measured routinely.

Renal disease is much the commonest cause of serious hypertension and will be diagnosed rapidly by the measurement of plasma urea and creatinine concentrations. Where these are normal, and especially if the serum potassium concentration is low, it will be reasonable to consider the endocrine causes of hypertension (Table 6.1). The hypertension of Turner

Table 6.1. *Endocrine causes of hypertension*

Congenital adrenal hyperplasia
   11β-hydroxylase deficiency
   17α-hydroxylase deficiency
Hyperaldosteronism
   Primary
   Dexamethasone suppressible
Cushing syndrome
Catecholamine excess

syndrome is more often renal than due to coarctation in my experience and I recommend that all Turner patients have renal investigations at least with ultrasound and possibly with isotopes.

The two varieties of congenital adrenal hyperplasia involved in the causation of hypertension affect sexual differentiation and development. 11β-hydroxylase deficiency is certainly likely to present with ambiguous genitalia in a girl and precocious puberty in a boy. The diagnosis has been discussed previously (Chapter 5) but it is worth stressing that the hypertension may be a late feature. Its treatment is to replace gluco-corticoid secretion: as previously indicated, the extent of the defect in aldosterone biosynthesis may be so severe that removal of CRH-ACTH drive may precipitate salt loss. Renin–angiotensin drive may then perpetuate hypertension and mineralocorticoid supplementation may be the answer in this situation.

17α hydroxylase deficiency causes ambiguity of the genitalia in males and failure of puberty in both sexes. The block may be so severe as to prevent male sexual differentiation altogether. As with 11β hydroxylase deficiency, hypertension (characterized by hypokalemia) may be a later presenting feature. The treatment is with glucocorticoid replacement but puberty will need attention.

Primary hyperaldosteronism is very rare in children. It may be due to bilateral adrenal hyperplasia or to an aldosterone producing tumour (as in adults). The treatment for the former is with spironolactone and surgery for the latter.

Dexamethasone suppressible hyperaldosteronism presents as hyper-aldosteronism (hypokalemia, hypertension, hyporeninemia and hyper-aldosteronemia) but has the characteristic feature of its name. Gluco-corticoid replacement controls the hypertension so a dexamethasone suppression test is needed in all children with hyperaldosteronism.

Cushing syndrome has been considered in Chapter 5. The hypertension may be severe and may persist after treatment owing to secondary changes.

Adrenomedullary hypertension, which may be episodic or sustained, is usually due to a tumour of neural crest origin such as pheochromocytoma, neuroblastoma or ganglioneuroma. There may be an association with other endocrine neoplasia (MEN2). Diagnosis requires measurement of blood catecholamines and/or their urinary metabolites and localization of their origin. Treatment requires surgical removal in the presence of an experienced anaesthetist and a carefully prepared (blocked) patient.

Water balance

Water balance is maintained by the action of the hypothalamic thirst centre in conjunction with the cerebral cortex controlling intake and hypothalamic osmoreceptors and neurones, which secrete arginine vaso-pressin (AVP or antidiuretic hormone, ADH), controlling output. The effect of AVP on water balance through its action in the collecting duct is truly remarkable. A child weighing 30 kg needs to excrete a solute load of about 800 mosmol/24 h: at the extreme of urinary dilution (50 mosmol/kg), this load could be excreted in 16 litres, at the extreme of concentration (1100 mosmol/kg) in 727 ml.

AVP and a larger polypeptide, a neurophysin, are synthesized in the supraoptic nuclei, the axonal processes of which form the supra-opticohypophyseal tract. The AVP–neurophysin complex, which prevents release of AVP by diffusion, forms granules that move along the axon to the neurohypophysis (posterior pituitary) for storage and release. Dilution and the higher pH in the bloodstream cause dissociation of the AVP–neurophysin complex.

Plasma AVP is related to plasma osmolality in a linear fashion with AVP secretion low enough at a plasma osmolality around 275 mosmol/kg to permit maximal urinary dilution. Urine osmolality is related to plasma AVP concentration in a logarithmic fashion: thus a 1 % change in plasma osmolality will produce an increase in plasma AVP of 1 pg/ml which will increase urinary osmolality by 250 mosmol/kg. Around a plasma osmolality of 295 mosmol/kg, AVP concentrations are sufficient to produce maximal urinary concentration. The threshold for thirst is about 10 mosmol/kg higher than those for AVP release so thirst is not usually perceived until plasma AVP levels are high enough to produce near maximal antidiuresis: the range of plasma osmolality in normal people is very narrow between 280 and 295 mosmol/kg.

Diagnosis, management and treatment of AVP deficiency

When AVP function is impaired, water is lost through the kidney and if thirst mechanisms are intact, the water lost will be replaced by drinking, the syndrome called diabetes insipidus (DI). The causes are shown in Table 6.2. A compulsive urge to drink is a not uncommon behavioural disorder in even very young children. If sufficient dilution is maintained for long enough, the kidney loses its medullary hyperosmolality and its ability to concentrate urine and it can be very difficult, especially in older patients, to distinguish compulsive water drinking from true AVP deficiency.

Because of the power of AVP to conserve water, a loss of more than 80 % of secretory capacity is required to become evident as DI. Thus it develops when a high proportion of the supraoptic neurones have been destroyed or when the pituitary stalk is severed above the pituitary diaphragm but not when the posterior pituitary alone is destroyed. There is an interaction between glucocorticoid secretion and the action of AVP so that in conditions of steroid lack the ability to excrete a water load is diminished. This explains the hyponatremia of isolated glucocorticoid deficiency. A lesion damaging the hypothalamo-pituitary area may cause AVP and ACTH deficiency, but the effect of the former may not become obvious until the latter is corrected by steroid replacement, which may then appear to trigger the symptoms of DI.

AVP deficiency is usually due to a tumour, its surgical treatment, trauma or a congenital abnormality of the hypothalamo-pituitary axis (Table 6.2). The search for a tumour must be prolonged and repeated: my personal record between the onset of symptoms and the final demonstration of a germinoma is 15 years. If AVP deficiency is associated with other pituitary hormone deficiencies, the chances of not finding a tumour are very small but it may be very difficult to find. Organ-specific antibodies against AVP producing cells have been shown in a few patients. Autosomal dominant and X-linked forms of AVP deficiency have been described but are very rare. The autosomal recessive association with diabetes mellitus, optic atrophy and deafness (DIDMOAD syndrome) occurs more frequently. DI should never be assumed to be idiopathic in children.

The symptoms of DI are usually unmistakable and of sudden onset but the degree of polyuria depends not only on the degree of AVP deficiency but also on the threshold for thirst and the osmolar load to be excreted. The diagnosis is established by demonstrating a discrepancy between the serum osmolality and a contemporaneous urine osmolality. *It is not necessary always to undertake a water deprivation test* and such a test can be

Table 6.2. *Causes of diabetes insipidus*

AVP deficiency
  Congenital abnormalities of the hypothalamo-pituitary axis
    e.g. septo-optic dysplasia
      midline defects
  Traumatic
    e.g. after intracranial surgery
      traumatic transection of the pituitary stalk (road traffic
        accidents)
  Inflammatory
    e.g. postmeningitis, especially in neonates
  Infiltrative
    e.g. histiocytosis
      sarcoid
  Tumours
    e.g. germinoma
      optic nerve glioma
      craniopharyngioma
  Autoimmune
  Genetic

Nephrogenic DI
  Sex-linked
  Associated with renal abnormalities
  Iatrogenic

---

dangerous in a severely AVP deficient patient. Fluids should never be withheld overnight in a patient with suspected DI. If a water deprivation test is required, it should be carried out under carefully observed conditions and after cortisol sufficiency has been assured.

When AVP deficiency has been confirmed, desmopressin (D-amino, D-arginine vasopressin, DDAVP) should be administered on a daily basis intranasally, the dose and its frequency being titrated against urine output and symptoms of thirst. Its adequacy can be checked using measurements of plasma osmolality but this is not usually required unless there is a concomitant lack of perception of thirst, which sometimes occurs in cases of DI following surgery and very occasionally in association with brain tumours.

DDAVP should never be given under any circumstances on the basis of either urinary output alone or values of urinary osmolality without corresponding plasma values, and especially not after surgery until the mismatch between plasma and urine osmolality has been unequivocally demonstrated. This is because the perioperative fluid replacement and steroid therapy can mimic DI; the administration of DDAVP to such a patient can cause water intoxication.

Long term management of DI requires continuous administration of DDAVP and free access to water. The dose of DDAVP required and its frequency varies considerably between individuals; in an individual patient it does also vary from time to time and upper respiratory tract infections and perennial or seasonal rhinitis can cause problems with intranasal administration. DDAVP has been given enterally and parenterally but a useful alternative to intranasal administration is to put the dose sublingually. Any patient with DI must be followed up to determine the onset or progression of other hypothalamo-pituitary hormone deficiencies, especially if the cause has not been elucidated.

In a patient who lacks perception of thirst, it is necessary to impose a strict regimen of fluid intake, then to replace AVP and then to check plasma osmolalities several times in a day. The combination of AVP and thirst deficiency is difficult for patient and physician. A patient with DI on treatment with DDAVP who has an intact thirst perception should never be forced to drink. Such patients cannot switch off endogenous AVP secretion like normal individuals and can become water intoxicated; this does not happen to normal patients which is why DDAVP has been found to be safe for use in normal children with nocturnal enuresis.

Diagnosis, management and treatment of nephrogenic diabetes insipidus

Two types of disease have been recognized, one with total resistance to the action of AVP and one requiring high concentrations of AVP to produce antidiuresis. Nephrogenic DI is inherited as a sex-linked recessive trait, but other conditions may impair the renal action of AVP, such as hypokalemia, hypercalcemia, sickle cell disease, polycystic kidneys, obstructive uropathy and chronic renal failure. A number of drugs, particularly cytotoxic therapy, may impair the action of AVP.

Treatment in complete AVP resistant states requires free access to water, but glomerular filtration can be reduced and the symptoms eased by a diet which controls the amount of solute to be excreted, by reducing glomerular filtration through the use of potassium sparing diuretics to induce mild dehydration and by inhibiting prostaglandin synthesis to enhance the effects of AVP. Drugs such as indomethacin also reduce glomerular filtration.

Diagnosis, management and treatment of AVP excess

The syndrome of inappropriate secretion of AVP leads to serum hypo-osmolality, hyponatremia, inappropriately high urinary osmolality and sodium loss. Plasma AVP levels are not usually elevated but are inappropriate for the serum osmolality. AVP may be secreted independently of osmolality or at an inappropriate osmolar threshold. Some tumours actually secrete AVP.

Excessive AVP release occurs in patients of all ages. It may follow any brain disease, including trauma and infection, especially in premature infants, lung disorders, such as pneumonia, and malignant disease and its treatment. It may be caused by drugs, including cytotoxic therapy, and occurs especially after narcotics and analgesics so it follows burns and surgery.

The symptoms may be headaches and apathy progressing to nausea, vomiting, abnormal neurological signs and impaired consciousness. In very severe cases there may be coma convulsions and death so this is not a situation to be taken lightly. Edema is not a feature of AVP excess because free water is evenly distributed in all body fluid compartments.

Treatment is to restrict fluid intake and to replace sodium lost secondarily. When extracellular expansion has been corrected, renal wastage of sodium will cease. Water intake then needs to be matched with output and this may be difficult to achieve in the presence of inappropriate thirst. In such a situation, drugs which inhibit AVP secretion may be effective.

7

Calcium balance

Clinical physiology

Vitamin D and its active metabolites, parathyroid hormone (PTH) and calcitonin, are the principal regulators of calcium metabolism. When plasma calcium falls, PTH release leads immediately to decreased renal calcium excretion and, in conjunction with 1,25-dihydroxyvitamin D, mobilization of calcium from bone. A slower action is to promote calcium and phosphate absorption from the gut. An undesirable rise in plasma phosphate concentration is prevented by the phosphaturic effect of PTH. Hypercalcemia inhibits PTH which leads to increased calcium excretion, decreased bone resorption and suppression of calcium binding in the gut. Serum phosphate concentrations are less strictly controlled; phosphate loss increases Vitamin D synthesis independently of PTH and phosphate retention inhibits it.

Vitamin D_3, cholecalciferol, is produced in the skin as a result of exposure of 7-dehydrocholesterol to ultraviolet light via a previtamin D_3 which undergoes slow conversion to cholecalciferol at body temperature. This has a high affinity for the Vitamin D binding protein, an α_2-globulin synthesized in the liver, whereas the previtamin remains in the skin. An excess of sunlight converts previtamin D_3 to inactive compounds thus preventing Vitamin D intoxication after sunbathing. Vitamin D may also be ingested and absorbed with chylomicrons. The concentration of the Vitamin D binding protein far exceeds the requirement for Vitamin D transport and it thereby acts as a reservoir supplying free Vitamin D metabolites to the cells.

Cholecalciferol is biologically inert and is 25-hydroxylated in the liver. A second hydroxylation occurs in the mitochondria of the proximal renal tubular cells; a number of compounds may be formed depending on the calcium requirement. 1,25-dihydroxycholecalciferol is the most active metabolite but 24,25-and 25,26-dihydroxycholecalciferol and other compounds with weak actions are also made but their biological function is not known.

1,25-dihydroxycholecalciferol binds to cell receptors and induces the synthesis of mRNA and the transcription of proteins which increase plasma calcium concentrations by stimulating intestinal absorption through the elaboration of a calcium binding protein and osteoclastic bone resorption. Whether the hormone has a direct effect on tubular function is unclear but it has a feedback mechanism on 1α-hydroxylation and is also a potent inhibitor of PTH secretion, the main effect of which is to increase 1α-hydroxylation. GH, prolactin and insulin also increase 1,25-dihydroxy Vitamin D synthesis. The concentration of 25-hydroxy-cholecalciferol is about 75 nmol/l and of 1,25-dihydroxycholecalciferol about 75 pmol/l, one-thousandth of the concentration, but the free levels of 1,25- are about one-tenth of the amount of free 25-OHD.

The gene for PTH is on chromosome 11. Active PTH is cleaved from a prohormone and secreted by the parathyroid glands in a response to plasma calcium concentration which is sigmoid shaped. Below a concentration of 2.0 mmol/l, PTH is maximally stimulated but it is not totally suppressed even by very high levels of plasma calcium concentration. Cortisol, prolactin, phosphate and vitamin D concentrations *inter alia* affect PTH secretion.

PTH has actions on the kidney to promote calcium reabsorption in the distal tubule and inhibition of phosphate and bicarbonate reabsorption in the proximal tubule where it also stimulates 1α-hydroxylation of 25-OHD. PTH stimulates osteoblasts to produce a factor which activates osteoclasts to mobilize calcium.

Calcitonin is produced by the C-cells of the thyroid gland. It is encoded by a gene on chromosome 11 and synthesized as a larger precursor molecule. The calcitonin gene also encodes a transcript in certain tissues which translates into calcitonin gene related peptide (CGRP) which is a very potent vasodilator. The role of calcitonin in regulating calcium metabolism is not clear. Its primary function seems to be to inhibit bone resorption by PTH and Vitamin D but it probably also has complex interactions with gastrointestinal hormones to prevent postprandial hypercalcemia.

Hypocalcemia

Most abnormalities of calcium and phosphorus can be explained by increased or decreased activity of $1,25 (OH)_2D$ or of PTH or by disordered kidney function. The clinician needs to have access to measurements of serum calcium, phosphate, alkaline phosphatase, creatinine, PTH, 25-OHD and $1,25-(OH)_2D$. He may need urinary measurements of calcium, phosphate, creatinine and cyclic AMP.

Neonatal hypocalcemia

Early neonatal hypocalcemia (within 72 hours of birth) is much the commonest problem in clinical practice and the one about which the least is known. Symptoms in the newborn are non-specific and include irritability, jitteriness and apnoea so the measurement of plasma calcium forms part of the routine biochemical screen. The main cause is attributed to cessation of placental supply of calcium, but PTH resistance and hypercalcitoninemia have also been postulated. It is important to remember that magnesium is required for the release but not for the synthesis of PTH, and hypomagnesemia is not uncommon, especially in the infants of diabetic mothers.

Hypocalcemia presenting later in the newborn period (4–28 days) is usually attributable to transient hypoparathyroidism or a high phosphate intake, but it may also be due to hypomagnesemia (especially in association with exposure to gentamicin), congenital hypoparathyroidism, malabsorption of calcium or maternal vitamin D deficiency.

Hypocalcemia in infants can be corrected in the emergency situation using 10% calcium gluconate intravenously. This is a poor source of oral calcium and calcium lactate is preferred for maintenance therapy. It is rarely necessary to resort to treatment with vitamin D preparations in the neonate.

Hypocalcemia in older patients

The symptoms of tetany (paraesthesiae, muscle cramps and weakness, carpopedal spasm and laryngospasm) are unmistakable as are the signs (Chvostek and Trousseau) but fits indistinguishable from epilepsy of any type may be the first feature of hypocalcemia. Indeed, epilepsy unresponsive to conventional medication should be assumed to have a (correctable) metabolic cause until proved otherwise. Since chronic hypocalcemia leads to mental retardation,cataracts and dental enamel problems, the diagnosis needs excluding early. A confusing issue can be hyperventilation and the resulting respiratory alkalosis which lowers ionized calcium but the total serum calcium will be normal.

In a patient who is hypocalcemic, a low serum phosphate concentration suggests that the cause is a form of phosphate losing rickets. A high phosphate concentration suggests hypoparathyroidism. A normal phosphate concentration indicates calciopenic rickets, the diagnosis of which is confirmed by an elevated serum alkaline phosphatase concentration and characteristic radiographic changes.

Rickets

The causes of rickets are shown in Table 7.1. Malabsorption of calcium and vitamin D are much more frequent than dietary deficiency, unless access to sunlight is also restricted, as may be the case in northern climes, in patients with dark skins and in ethnic groups who wear closely protective clothing for religious reasons. The theory that some sorts of chapati flour bind calcium and vitamin D seems to have lost currency recently.

Decreased vitamin D dependent calcium absorption induces hypocalcemia and secondary hyperparathyroidism, which leads in turn to increased phosphate excretion and hypophosphatemia. Diminished calcium and phosphate levels cause defective bone mineralization (bone softening and bending), and secondary hyperparathyroidism causes increased bone resorption (swollen metaphyses), the combination accounting for the clinical, histological and radiological findings of rickets. Bone pain and muscle weakness are common and retard motor milestones but the most striking clinical feature is growth retardation or stand-still.

Malabsorption is a feature of severe liver disease, but there may also be a diminution in the 25-hydroxylation of cholecalciferol which must be remembered when it comes to treating the calciopenic rickets of liver disease. Anticonvulsant medication may inhibit gastrointestinal absorption of calcium and vitamin D but also induces hepatic enzyme systems leading to increased catabolism of vitamin D metabolites.

Defects in vitamin D synthesis were associated with the need for high levels of Vitamin D replacement in therapy, hence the term Vitamin D dependent rickets which should be abandoned on the grounds of imprecision. 1α-hydroxylation deficiency may be an inborn error but it can also accompany progressive loss of nephrons in renal disease. In that situation, there is also phosphate retention which is the primary cause of

Table 7.1. *Causes of rickets*

Calciopenic
    Calcium deficiency
        – dietary
        – malabsorption
    Vitamin D deficiency
        – dietary
        – malabsorption
        – no sunlight
        – liver disease
        – associated with anticonvulsant medication
    Biosynthetic defect of Vitamin D
        – 1α-hydroxylase deficiency
        – liver disease
        – renal disease
    Defective action of Vitamin D
        – receptor binding deficiency, partial or complete
        – failure of translocation to nucleus
        – transcription defects
        – posttranscription defects

Phosphopenic
    Renal tubular loss of phosphate
        – isolated defect
            X-linked hypophosphatemic rickets
            Autosomal recessive and dominant forms
        – mixed tubular disorders
            Fanconi syndrome
            Oculo-cerebro-renal syndrome
            nephrotoxic agents
            renal tubular acidosis
    Decreased phosphate intake

Abnormal bones
    Hypophosphatasia
    Renal osteodystrophy

renal osteodystrophy; this can be assisted by restricting dietary phosphate, which improves calcium absorption through an increase in 1,25-$(OH)_2D$. End organ defects of vitamin D are inherited in an autosomal recessive fashion and such patients need very large doses of 1,25-dihydroxy vitamin D.

Phosphate-losing rickets often presents simply with short stature. As this is most frequently the sex-linked recessive disease, males are more severely affected than the heterozygote females. The severity of the bone deformity varies widely and does not seem to be linked to the severity of the biochemical findings. Classically these patients are normocalcemic, but this is certainly not always the case, and hypocalcemia may be seen both in the untreated patient and after phosphate replacement. Ectopic calcification does occur in untreated adult patients, but is a serious complication of treatment with the phosphate used to promote normal growth in these children, vitamin D being used to prevent hypocalcemia.

X-linked hypophosphatemic rickets must be distinguished from the other causes of phosphopenic rickets shown in Table 7.1, but the renal problems usually present with other symptoms before those of rickets.

Treatment of rickets requires calcium, phosphate and Vitamin D in varying combinations to correct clinical, radiological and biochemical abnormalities. Growth assessment is a powerful tool for detecting the success of therapy; as serum alkaline phosphatase reflects bone turnover, which is what growth requires, following the concentration of this to determine progress may not be helpful. A careful watch on serum calcium and phosphate concentrations on any therapy is needed. In vitamin D deficiency, the safest treatment is with cholecalciferol and additional calcium if hypocalcemia is, or becomes, a feature in the individual patient. For patients with rickets secondary to defects in vitamin D synthesis or action, or associated with other disorders, 25-hydroxycholecalciferol, 1α-hydroxycholecalciferol or 1,25-dihydroxycholecalciferol may be used with respective increasing potency and decreasing half life.

Hypoparathyroidism

An embryonal defect resulting in absence or hypoplasia of the parathyroid glands presents with hypocalcemia in the newborn period. The association of hypoparathyroid deficiency with thymic abnormalities, cardiac defects and facial abnormalities (diGeorge syndrome) is often not complete. It is usually sporadic but may be autosomal dominant or recessive. Hypoparathyroidism in older children is usually autoimmune and may be associated with other autoimmune diseases, mucocutaneous candidiasis, Addison disease and hypothyroidism. Hypoparathyroidism may also follow thyroid surgery, even if the surgeon is certain that the parathyroid glands have been identified and preserved.

Hypocalcemia and hyperphosphatemia resistant to parathyroid extract was called pseudohypoparathyroidism by Albright in 1942. Most patients are mentally retarded and they have short stature, a characteristic face and shortening of the metacarpal and metatarsal bones as a result of premature fusion of the epiphyses. Ectopic calcification and ossification is common. The diagnosis is suggested by the finding of PTH concentrations elevated disproportionately to the serum calcium, and can be confirmed by the failure to increase urinary cyclic AMP when the stimulus of PTH is applied. In many such patients, TSH concentrations are raised, although T_4 may be normal suggesting TSH resistance. It is usual to treat such patients with thyroxine as well as the calcium and Vitamin D required to prevent the symptoms of hypocalcemia and its consequences.

Patients with the phenotype of what has been called Albright's hereditary osteodystrophy without biochemical evidence of renal resistance to PTH have pseudopseudohypoparathyroidism. What exactly is wrong with them has not been elucidated.

Treatment of patients with hypoparathyroidism or pseudohypoparathyroidism requires calcium and vitamin D. The serum calcium has an irritating tendency to fluctuate even though there appears to be no reason to explain the fluctuations. Hypercalcemia is undesirable because it leads to hypercalciuria and stone formation; for this reason it is easier to use vitamin D preparations with a short half-life so that an elevated calcium concentration can quickly be returned to normal.

Hypercalcemia

Anorexia, constipation, polyuria, nausea and vomiting are such non-specific symptoms within a pattern of failure to thrive that the diagnosis of hypercalcemia may very easily be overlooked. In a patient with persistent hypercalcemia, the measurement of serum PTH concentration is very useful. The concentration will be low in vitamin D intoxication, in infantile hypercalcemia and in association with tumours but high in primary hyperparathyroidism and in familial hypocalciuric hypercalcemia. Since the latter is a benign condition and the former needs surgical treatment, the separation of them by the measurement of urinary calcium excretion (raised in hyperparathyroidism and normal or low in hypocalciuric hypercalcemia) is important. Unfortunately this may call for metabolic ward conditions to measure calcium intake as well as output.

Stone formation occurs whenever there is hypercalciuria. Most frequently this accompanies hypercalcemia but it may result from increased intestinal calcium absorption secondary either to increased vitamin D concentrations or to increased responsiveness to normal levels. The former is usually iatrogenic and responds to alterations in therapy; the latter requires dietary calcium restriction.

Hypercalcemia in infancy comes in two forms. There is a mild form which presents with severe feeding difficulties but runs a benign and self-limiting course over the first year of life. There is a more serious form associated with a typical facies, dysmorphic features, mental retardation and cardiovascular anomalies, classically aortic stenosis (Williams syndrome). Some patients with Williams syndrome do not have hypercalcemia.

There is no way certainly to distinguish the two forms of hypercalcemia if the dysmorphic features are not obvious except by the passage of time. The remedy, therefore, is to limit dietary calcium and vitamin D intake in both and to hope for the best outcome. In emergency, hypercalcemia responds to administration of glucocorticoids (prednisolone) and copious fluids.

Hyperparathyroidism is not common in children but it is a part of multiple endocrine neoplasia (MEN) types I (with gastrinoma and pituitary tumours) and II (with medullary thyroid cancer and phaeochromocytoma). Children from affected families should be screened for hypercalcemia. The diagnosis of hyperparathyroidism requires the demonstration of hypercalcemia and persistent elevation of PTH concentration. The main differential diagnosis in children is from benign familial hypocalciuric hypercalcemia because PTH levels can also be elevated in this condition. The way to make the distinction is by demonstrating a low calcium excretion in relation to the hypercalcemia (it is elevated in hyperparathyroidism), which can be done by comparing the ratio of calcium clearance to creatinine clearance which will be lower than 0.01 in the benign condition. Parathyroid adenomata, which account for 80% of cases of hyperparathyroidism in adults, are very uncommon in children, but parathyroid hyperplasia does occur and requires surgical treatment.

8

Glucose homeostasis

The concentration of glucose in the blood is the result of a balance between food intake and glucose mobilization from the liver, on the one hand, and its consumption by the tissues on the other. The former is regulated by many hormones but the latter only by insulin.

During feeding, increased blood glucose and amino acid levels, as well as gut hormones, stimulate insulin secretion from the cells of the pancreas. The main action of insulin is in the liver where it stimulates conversion of glucose to glycogen and decreases gluconeogenesis and glycogenolysis. The liver consumes much of the insulin secreted so that an assessment of endogenous insulin secretion into the portal vein has to be made by the measurement of plasma C (connecting) peptide concentrations in peripheral blood. C peptide is split from pro-insulin in equimolar amounts but is not removed by the liver. The insulin which gets through the liver is diluted in the extracellular volume but still exerts profound peripheral effects stimulating uptake of glucose and amino acids by muscle and of glucose by fat cells to form triglyceride.

During fasting, the blood glucose concentration falls, insulin production reduces under the influence of pancreatic somatostatin and glucagon is secreted by the pancreatic α cells. The falling glucose level is sensed in the hypothalamus which regulates pancreatic secretion by neural mechanisms and stimulates release of ACTH (and thereby cortisol), GH, prolactin and catecholamines. These counter-regulatory mechanisms inhibit glucose uptake and stimulate amino acid release by muscle; they promote lipolysis and release of free fatty acids from adipose tissue and induce glycogenolysis and gluconeogenesis in the liver. The production of ketones in the fasting state results from lipolysis and subsequent hepatic fatty acid β-oxidation.

Diabetes mellitus

General overview

There is a huge geographical variation in the incidence of diabetes in children up to the age of 15 years; recent figures range from 4.6 cases per 100000 per year in northern Greece to 42.9 in Finland. The comparable figure for UK is 16.5 with a slight excess of males and a considerable increase in the number of cases diagnosed over 10 years of age compared to 0–4 and 5–9.

The cause of diabetes is not known, except that some genetically susceptible individuals have islet cell antibodies which destroy the β-cells of the pancreas. An enormous effort has been devoted to determining the environmental triggers of the autoimmune process, which has been fuelled by the geographical differences in incidence. An effort of similar magnitude has been directed at predicting the onset of diabetes in first degree relatives of diabetic patients with the intention of delaying or preventing the onset of the disease. So far, neither effort has achieved real success. Efforts of similar magnitude and lack of success have also been directed towards the preservation of insulin production after the diagnosis of diabetes mellitus has been established.

Diabetes mellitus is not a disorder of sudden onset. There is a progressive loss of islet cell function at a variable rate which may take a lifetime to reach the stage of decompensation between glucose input and insulin secretion which manifests itself as clinical diabetes. For this reason, type 1 diabetes can present at any age from infancy to the ninth decade and the symptoms may be more or less insidious depending upon the rate at which decompensation is reached.

Initially there is nearly always some endogenous insulin secretory activity remaining so a replacement regimen provides a background insulin level against which fine control is exerted endogenously (the 'honeymoon' period), but progressive loss of islet cells leads to the irreversible dependency on exogenous insulin.

When insulin production fails, the effect can be predicted. The blood glucose rises and the glucose in the glomerular filtrate exceeds the ability of the proximal tubules to reabsorb it which leads to glycosuria. The resulting osmolality of the contents of the renal tubule prevents the counter-current mechanisms from concentrating the urine in the loop of Henle because the renal medulla is insufficiently hyperosmolar. The distal tubular and collecting duct mechanisms for conserving free water fail and its loss presents as polyuria. The contraction of extracellular volume leads to thirst and polydipsia. When the extracellular volume becomes severely depleted, the end diastolic filling pressure falls and the cardiac output drops.

Initial management

The first requirement for the treatment of acute diabetes is fluid to restore circulating blood volume. This cannot be given as the water which has been lost (in practice this would be as its isosmotic equivalent) because there is intracellular dehydration and the result of quickly lowering extracellular osmolality would be intracellular edema. In fact, imaging has shown that ventricular size becomes compressed during the treatment of acute ketoacidosis with saline in most subjects, which implies a degree of cerebral edema, but severe cerebral edema is greatly to be feared since it is the commonest cause of death in children with acute diabetes. This is why it is best to hurry slowly in the treatment of acute ketoacidosis, aiming to restore homeostasis over 48 h.

When insulin levels are low, as they are in the Type 1, insulin-dependent diabetes seen in children, liver glycogen is mobilized to glucose; muscle protein is mobilized to free amino acids; adipose tissue triglyceride is mobilized to free fatty acids; β-oxidation metabolizes free fatty acids to ketone bodies. The result is the ketoacidosis of uncontrolled insulin deficiency. Since potassium enters cells with glucose, extracellular potassium concentrations may rise. All these events can be controlled by the administration of insulin.

Management of ketoacidosis

Insulin action is determined by the number and affinity of insulin receptors: these are inversely related to the concentration of circulating insulin so the sudden administration of a large bolus defeats its object because of tissue down regulation of receptors. This is the reason why quick-acting soluble insulin should be given by slow intravenous infusion for the treatment of severe ketoacidosis.

Emergency management of acute diabetic ketoacidosis thus comprises:

1. Intravenous saline given at a rate of 20 ml/kg/h over the first hour to restore extracellular fluid volume. The total fluid deficiency is probably around 100 ml/kg and this should be replaced in addition to continuing losses and metabolic requirements over the next 48 h at a rate of about 10 ml/kg/h. 5% dextrose should be

added to the infusate as the blood glucose concentration falls to around 10 mmol/l (which it will do slowly without insulin but more quickly with it).

2. Intravenous soluble insulin initially at a dose of 0.05 IU/kg/h if the blood glucose concentration is less than 15 mmol/l and 0.1 IU/kg/h if it exceeds this. A loading bolus is contraindicated for the reasons explained above. The rate of infusion should be assessed and adjusted by measuring blood glucose concentration hourly until it is changing by less than 3 mmol/h, and then 2 hourly.

As well as monitoring glucose, serum potassium concentrations should be checked at 2–4 hourly intervals, and replacement given if necessary at a rate of 2 mmol/kg/24 h. The metabolic acidosis will correct itself but, if the initial pH is less than 7.1, sodium bicarbonate may be added to the infusate in a dose of 10% of the base deficit/kg/24 h until the pH has risen above 7.1. Careful monitoring should prevent hypoglycemia, hypokalemia, hypernatremia and, most importantly, cerebral edema.

Long-term management

It is an act of faith that the normalization of blood glucose concentrations in diabetic patients will prevent or delay the onset of the microvascular, ocular, neurological and nephrological complications of longstanding type-1 diabetes. Since good control leading to long term lowering of glycated hemoglobin concentrations has a beneficial impact on the progression of non-proliferative retinopathy, although it does not prevent its development, the aim of most physicians is to try to normalize blood glucose levels in diabetic children.

Unfortunately, they rarely if ever succeed because insulin is given in the wrong place (systemically rather than into the portal circulation), at the wrong time (before meals rather than during or after them) and induces the wrong serum concentration profile because the injections are given subcutaneously even if they are given very frequently. A multiple injection or infusion regimen is not tolerated by most children so combinations of long and shorter acting insulins are used to enable the use of twice daily injection regimens.

Because insulin is given before food (about 30 minutes is best, less if the injection is into central adipose tissue rather than limbs), the food has to be tailored to the insulin which has been administered rather than the other way round which is how normal people regulate their insulin secretion.

This is one of the reasons for attention to diet in diabetic children. The other reasons include:

1. the need to have complex carbohydrates to slow absorption of glucose to match the unphysiological profile of insulin generated by a subcutaneous injection;
2. the need to eat frequently and at regular intervals for the same reason;
3. the belief that a low fat diet is effective in delaying or preventing the progression of atherosclerosis to which diabetic patients are especially prone because of the effect of their insulin deficiency on adipose tissue metabolism. Since hypertension is the major determinant of atherosclerotic cardiovascular disease, and diabetic patients are prone to this because of the renal complications, the low fat diet should also be low in salt.

Ideally then, a diabetic child should have:

1. adequate protein;
2. small amounts of fat;
3. complex carbohydrate usually associated with fibre to provide over 50 and preferably nearer to 55% of the dietary calorie requirements.

In practice, this translates to lean meats and, better, fish and poultry. Dairy products, eggs, margarine and oil should be limited. Sugar, honey, jam, sweets, sauces, soft drinks and cordials are to be avoided because they cause the blood glucose to rise rapidly in a way that the exogenously induced insulin profile cannot meet. Wholegrain bread and cereals, wholemeal pasta, brown rice, fruit and vegetables with the skin if possible are strongly to be encouraged. It is all fairly obvious but, of course, few children will stick to such a list.

The long-term management of diabetes thus becomes a compromise between an undesirable insulin regimen and unacceptable dietary restriction. Current modes of therapy rarely, if ever, normalize blood glucose levels, and the diabetic suffers not only a restriction of lifestyle but also the inevitability of complications and a life expectancy which has not changed with the change seen in the normal population.

A charge of therapeutic nihilism might be levelled against the author of the preceding paragraph – and this author actually believes in the aim of normalizing blood glucose concentrations in the diabetic child. It is my belief derived from long observation, however, that most multidisciplinary teams caring for diabetic children have forgotten the size of the task which

Table 8.1. *Types of insulin*

	Start of action	Peak action	End of effect	Danger of hypoglycemia
Quick acting (neutral/soluble)	0.5 h	1–4 h	8 h	1–5 h
Moderately slow (NPH*/isophane)	1.5 h	4–12 h	24 h	8–18 h
Slow (insulin zinc suspensions)	4 h	6–18 h	24 h	12–20 h
Very slow (suspension of insulin crystals)	4 h	8–24 h	30 h	24 h

* NPH = Neutral protamine Hagedorn after the Danish scientist who discovered the delaying effect of attaching insulin to protamine.

they impose on their patients: they are ready to accuse them of 'non-compliance' and are inclined to focus attention on the dose of insulin and the reinforcement of 'education'. This is easy, what they understand and what they are trained to deliver; perhaps they need to acknowledge and make the best of what is an intolerable situation if the truth is to be told.

In practice, long term management of diabetes in children requires a regimen which includes:

1. a diet as near ideal as possible in quality; quantity should not be an issue and should be determined by the child. The problem is that once the quantity has been decided and the insulin titrated against it, that quantity has to be consumed day in, day out;
2. food intake which should be regular and as unvarying in time as possible;
3. insulin (Table 8.1) which should be given either twice daily or before each main meal and before bed (i.e. 4 times daily). In the former regimen, it is likely that a two-thirds : one-third mixture of long- and short-acting insulins will be required for each of the two injections, two-thirds of the total dose being given in the morning. In the latter regimen, a short acting insulin is used three times daily before main meals and a long acting insulin administered at bed time. The total amount of insulin needed depends, of course, upon the size of the patient but then, first, upon the degree of insulin deficiency which has been reached and, secondly, upon the other hormones circulating.

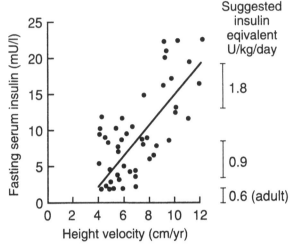

Fig. 8.1. Relation between fasting insulin concentrations and growth velocity in normal children together with guidelines for insulin doses required in diabetic children to give normal growth.

In paediatric practice, the main counter-regulatory hormone which is likely to be changing with age is growth hormone. This determines the rate of growth, so the rate of growth becomes related to fasting insulin concentrations in normal children (Fig. 8.1). The growth rate expected at any age can therefore be used to give an indication of insulin requirements in diabetic children. Since insulin is a major translator of the GH message in normal children, an insufficient dose of soluble insulin will retard the growth of diabetic children. This becomes especially obvious at puberty

4. The quantity and quality (duration of action) of insulin required should be tailored to the measurement of a blood glucose profile. Blood glucose measurements should not be a matter of routine record: if they provide no useful information to the patient, they are valueless and a sensible patient will not perform them. Home blood glucose monitoring is a considerable advance but it must be used to the advantage of the patient and not as a stick with which to beat him or her.

I recommend measuring blood glucose concentration in a diabetic patient either 4 hourly throughout 24 hours at weekly or two weekly intervals, depending on the stability of the condition or twice (or more) daily measurements at different times of the day on several days of the week to yield the same information. Values of blood glucose concentration during the night are particularly valuable since nocturnal hypoglycemia is strongly to be discouraged because it affects mental performance directly and also by disturbing sleep. On the other hand, lack of control at night will lead to progressive rise of glycosylated hemoglobin concentrations and poor control of diabetes overall.

Blood glucose profiles will provide information upon which therapeutic decisions can be made, and consequently they should be more likely to be performed rather than falsified, especially by adolescents.

Special problems

Injection technique and site are important to avoid fibro-fatty lumps which cause irregular insulin absorption. The use of disposable needles has been an improvement, but damage to underlying tissues can be lessened by avoiding swabbing the skin with alcohol before injection. Ordinary cleanliness is quite sufficient.

Skin infections, particularly paronychia, are common in diabetic children and the vicious cycle of staphylococcal infection and poor diabetic control may need vigorous measures to interrupt it. Limited joint mobility is a sign of poor control and/or duration of diabetes; its connection with micro-vascular changes is disputed.

Paediatricians need to keep abreast of research into the prevention of the complications of diabetes. Just because they are rarely seen in paediatric practice does not excuse a failure to look for them. Prevention should begin in childhood. Although prevention by controlling blood glucose concentrations has not been very effective, measurement of glucose excretion in the 24 h urine specimens collected to detect microalbuminuria can reveal an alarming discrepancy between real and apparent control and a serious loss of (carbohydrate) calories, which will affect growth or be made up by calories from fat, which will not be good for the arteries, or protein, which will not be good for the kidneys.

Assessment of long term control is practised widely using a measure of glucose binding to protein. Glycosylated hemoglobin concentration is as good as any other measure, but it must be remembered that falsely low values can be obtained if there are alternating periods of hyper- and hypoglycemia because the measurement is of a mean value. M-values (the cumulative deviations of the blood glucose concentration from its mean values) may be high and keep glycosylated hemoglobin concentrations artificially low. For this reason, home glucose monitoring cannot be abandoned in favour of measurements of long-term control.

Serum fructosamine measurement reflects glucose control over a shorter period than glycosylated hemoglobin and is dependent upon normal albumin kinetics. To yield information comparable to that derived from HbA_{1c} measurement, it would have to be measured more frequently and it is, therefore, not a satisfactory substitute, except in certain well defined situations such as pregnancy.

Complications of diabetes are usually not considered sufficiently by paediatricians. Macrovascular complications need early preventive measures to be taken. In the paediatric clinic, this means exposing the folly of smoking and assessing other risk factors, especially blood pressure and plasma cholesterol fractions, at regular intervals. Because hypothyroidism has a greatly increased incidence in diabetic patients, thyroid function should be measured from time to time and all diabetic patients should be screened for the presence of thyroid antibodies. Lipoprotein (a) may become increasingly important, especially if it can be confirmed that it is influenced by renal function and blood pressure, as seems likely.

Screening for complications should be part of the surveillance of diabetic children, and perhaps the only part where a physician is needed rather than other professionals. Just because complications are rarely seen in paediatric or adolescent patients does not absolve the physician from the search for them. Only paediatricians have the key to unravelling the natural history of diabetic complications but there is a real practical aspect because intensification of control measures does retard their progression.

Ideally, every child should be screened for the onset of complications of diabetes at annual intervals from the time of diagnosis. The problem is that not many clinics (especially in the UK) are big enough to justify the investment needed properly to undertake this task. There may be a place, therefore, for centralization of screening services for diabetic children, because it is certain that they cannot benefit from advances in prediction and prevention of the condition they already have. We have a duty to ensure that we make the best of their fate.

Screening involves:

- measurement of serum lipid fractions and lipoproteins;
- measurement of thyroid function;
- consideration of celiac disease and autoimmune disorders;
- ophthalmological examination;
- renal function tests;
- recording of blood pressure with random zero sphygmomanometer;

- tests of autonomic and peripheral nerve function;
- objective assessment of joint mobility.

Ophthalmological examination should be routine in the clinic but specialist examination is needed at regular intervals. This will include retinal photography and the facility for fluorescein angiography, as well as access to laser treatment. Good control of blood glucose concentrations will retard the progress of a retinopathy. Cataract is a complication of long-term poor control, and may be quite commonly seen in diabetic children and adolescents.

Renal failure is a common cause of death in older diabetics, and diabetes is the second most common cause of chronic renal failure. The initial problem is intermittent and then persistent microalbuminuria (20–200 micrograms/min). At this stage, the GFR and blood pressure are both normal. When albuminuria (Albustix positive) becomes evident, progression to diabetic nephropathy is inevitable, blood pressure rises and GFR falls. It should be remembered that spermaturia is common in adolescent boys, which may give false positive screening results. Orthostatic proteinuria may also cause confusion.

Efforts should be made to detect microalbuminuria early by annual timed overnight collections of urine. Blood pressure is related to albumin output and is slightly elevated in affected diabetic children. Whether increased blood pressure is the cause or effect of microalbuminuria, the use of age-specific blood pressure charts should be encouraged to detect it. It is probable that the increased glomerular filtration which causes microalbuminuria results from intraglomerular hypertension, which suggests a possibility for secondary prevention using antihypertensive therapy. The treatment of hypertension with ACE inhibitors may be particularly effective because renin substrate is elevated in diabetics with microalbuminuria. A rising level of prorenin may precede microalbuminuria, and its measurement may become a marker for the risk of both retinopathy and nephropathy.

It may become possible to treat young diabetics in the phase of preclinical nephropathy by lowering blood pressure and prorenin levels. This could delay the progress of the microalbuminuria to the overt proteinuria which precedes renal failure. It might also help lipoprotein (a) concentrations and so bear on the progress of macrovascular complications.

Autonomic dysfunction and peripheral neuropathy are tested by measuring heart rate changes to respiration and the Valsalva manoeuvre, by measuring blood pressure changes to posture, by assessing pupillary reaction times and by testing perception of temperature and vibration changes applied to the limbs. Neuropathies are not often observed in children but should be remembered because good control imposed at an early stage improves nerve conduction velocity and sensation of vibration. Loss of autonomic function becomes progressively irreversible.

Adolescence is a time of special problems. There is first the disruption which the hormonal changes of puberty bring to diabetic control. Growth hormone has an antiinsulin activity and consequently it is much more difficult to maintain stability of blood glucose when the hormone levels are changing. An increase in insulin to match growth rate is obviously one requirement but few adolescents who are totally insulin dependent get through this period of time with ease. Most experience swings of blood glucose concentration, high and low, which are not simple to explain. The physician needs to be humble – the expertise on offer is pretty limited – and understanding if the trust of the patient, who may well be feeling that not much help is forthcoming, is not to be forfeited. Blaming the patient for lack of control is not helpful, even if dietary indiscretion plays a major part in determining poor control in some individuals.

Adolescence is also the time when a child assumes responsibility for its own actions. The realization of what having diabetes as an adult really means in terms of restriction of lifestyle, work availability and the threat of complications may be very disturbing. The patient might well (and justifiably) feel cheated in the fact that, no matter what happens, major problems loom on the horizon because of the shadow of diabetes.

Adolescence is a two way process which requires action on the part of the parents, the physician and his (paediatric) team to disengage their involvement as well as action on the part of the child. This is always painful but never more so than in diabetes because of the (legitimate) concern which the parents and physician retain for the well-being of the child in the face of their increasing lack of control. There is no easy recipe for success but paediatricians at least can assist the process by discontinuing the attendance of adolescent diabetic patients to a children's clinic sooner rather than later. Whether they choose to set up specific clinics for adolescents, or joint clinics with physicians in adult practice, probably does not matter but the removal of an adolescent from a paediatric setting is an important contribution to the hard task the family has to achieve.

Brittle diabetes, the inability of a diabetic patient to live life without repeated episodes of ketoacidosis and/or hypoglycemia, is now widely recognized to have a psychological rather than a physical basis. The pursuit of blood glucose control without trying to resolve the underlying problem is especially futile in such instances; even though the resolution of that problem is a sisyphean task, it should be tackled – probably by a centre set up for the purpose.

Travel should not be a problem for the diabetic patient. When the travel is towards the west, additional injections of soluble insulin are required at 4 – 6 hourly intervals to accommodate the time changes. When the travel is towards the east, it is preferable to manage on frequent injections of soluble insulin and to reinstate the use of longer acting insulins on arrival according to the time change. Airlines are expert in supplying the necessary food intake. What they are not so good about is avoiding delays in travel schedules, and diabetic patients should be warned to expect them and be well supplied with snacks as well as insulin to deal with the difficulties they cause in blood glucose control.

Exercise is strongly to be encouraged in the diabetic patient but it needs, like food intake, to be regular to be easily accommodated into the diabetic therapeutic regimen and can cause still more problems for the patient. Adequate supplies of long-acting carbohydrate are especially important to such patients. They should also be advised to avoid injecting insulin into an exercising area (legs or arms), since the speed of absorption can be markedly altered from that to which they may have become accustomed. Physicians should be aware that insulin requirements can drop dramatically in those who are physically very active either in sport or otherwise (e.g. ballet dancers).

Hypoglycemia

Because of the balance which maintains a stable blood glucose concentration, the causes of hypoglycemia (Table 8.2) can be divided into those which cause inadequate mobilization of glucose into the blood, and those which are associated with excessive removal of glucose from it.

There is argument regarding the definition of hypoglycemia, some authorities defining it by the measurement of blood glucose concentrations (< 2.2 mmol/l or 40 mg/dl) and others requiring symptoms to establish a diagnosis. Because the symptoms are so protean (Table 8.3), a biochemical definition is to be preferred. Even so, in a neonate, there is little evidence to suggest that asymptomatic hypoglycemia is associated with permanent neurological damage and blood glucose concentrations can certainly approach the arbitrary level of 2.2 mmol/l in normal children after a prolonged fast without apparent damage.

Glucose utilization in normal infants ranges from 5 – 10 mg/kg/min and in adults is 2 mg/kg/min. Thus, in a patient with persistent

Table 8.2. *Causes of hypoglycemia*

Inadequate glucose production
Insufficient glycogen (usually transient and in the neonate)
Glycogen storage diseases
Enzyme deficiencies
e.g. Galactosemia, fructose intolerance and other metabolic defects
Hormone deficiencies
e.g. GH, ACTH, Glucocorticoids, glucagon, catecholamines
Liver disease
Alcohol
Salicylates
Excessive glucose consumption
Infant of diabetic mother
Beckwith–Wiedemann syndrome
Nesidioblastosis
Insulinoma
Factitious or excessive insulin administration
Oral hypoglycemic agents

Table 8.3. *Symptoms of hypoglycemia*

Neonate
Irritability
Feeding problems
Tremors and jitteriness
Apnoea
Hypotonia
Convulsions
Coma
Older patients
Lack of energy
Headaches and/or abdominal pain
Hunger
Pallor and sweating
Mental confusion
Behavioural abnormalities
Convulsions
Coma

hypoglycemia requiring a constant infusion of intravenous glucose, it is not difficult to decide whether the problem is due to inadequate glucose production or to excessive glucose utilization and take the appropriate route to define the diagnosis. However, energy stores as glycogen are limited to about 12 hours in the older child so it is not surprising that many neonates, especially premature ones, need very frequent feeds to avoid hypoglycemia. All illnesses increase metabolic demand and consequently increase the need for glucose.

Management

Much useful information can be derived by taking blood for biochemical estimations but *only if it is taken when the patient is actually hypoglycemic*. In such a situation, blood samples should be taken and stored for the later measurement of any or all of the following:

- blood glucose;
- insulin;
- cortisol;
- growth hormone;
- lactate;
- free fatty acids;
- amino acids;
- ketones;
- C-peptide.

Hypoglycemia in the absence of urinary ketones is likely to be due to excessive consumption of glucose (hyperinsulinemia), unless there is a defect in fatty acid β-oxidation which will be recognized by a discrepancy with the plasma levels of free fatty acids. Hypoglycemia with ketosis is likely to be due to hormone deficiencies or to enzyme deficiencies.

The measurement of blood lactate is intended to assist in the diagnosis of glycogen storage disorders but the definition of the type and its management is the province of a specialized centre. The measurement of amino acids will assist in the diagnosis of inborn errors of metabolism, and the same applies to diagnosis and management. Since insulin and C peptide are secreted in equimolar amounts, the finding of plasma insulin in the absence of C peptide suggests factitious administration of insulin.

Treatment

The administration of glucose intravenously is the fastest and safest way to relieve symptoms of hypoglycemia. It is not necessary and generally undesirable to use a concentration of glucose greater than 20% and most patients can be managed with glucose solutions less concentrated than this.

If there is difficulty in establishing an intravenous line and there are problems with enteral feeding, a subcutaneous injection of glucagon (0.1 mg/kg) will assist in controlling the hypoglycemia. Glucagon, however, stimulates insulin secretion; thus, although it is useful in the (insulin-dependent) diabetic patient, it may cause hyperinsulinism and reactive hypoglycemia in a patient with intact insulin secretion. It is also ineffective in a starved patient with glycogen depletion because there is no substrate for it to mobilize. In children with nesidioblastosis, somatostatin and its long-acting analogue may help in controlling insulin secretion and excessive glucose consumption.

9

The endocrine consequences of neoplasia

Hormone-secreting tumours are not common in children but tumours, particularly intracranial neoplasms, have effects on the endocrine system in general and the hypothalamo-pituitary axis in particular. Treatment with surgery, chemotherapy and radiotherapy has extensive consequences on the endocrine system.

Primary disorders

Leukemia is the commonest malignant disease in children. It rarely affects hormone secretion but its treatment frequently does so (see below). Intracranial space occupying lesions come second with an annual incidence of 2.2–2.5 brain tumours per 100000 children; supratentorial tumours are commoner in children under the age of 4 years and in adults but, in the age-group 4–11 years, infratentorial tumours outnumber supratentorial by 3 to 1.

Tumours in the posterior fossa (50%), lateral ventricles and cerebral hemispheres (30%) usually present with symptoms of raised intracranial pressure or a neurological complaint (e.g.epilepsy) and rarely with endocrine disorders. However, children with brain tumours in any situation grow badly and a diminution of growth velocity is often the first sign of tumour relapse, so whenever growth assessment reveals a problem, the possibility of a brain tumour distant from the hypothalamo-pituitary axis should be considered. Gonadotrophin-dependent (central) precocious puberty may be a consequence of simple hydrocephalus so any tumour may present in this way.

Tumours of the optic nerve, pituitary, pineal or hypothalamus, which comprise 20% of childhood intracranial neoplasms, may have direct endocrine effects on growth, usually inhibiting it, on pubertal development, causing it to be either early or late, or on thirst and appetite. Craniopharyngioma, optic nerve or hypothalamic glioma, pineal tumours and hamartoma are the tumour types most frequently associated with direct endocrine effects as a result of their position in the hypothalamo-pituitary axis.

Hormone secreting tumours include prolactinoma, which may cause galactorrhoea but usually affects pubertal onset; pheochromocytoma and carcinoid tumours, which present with hypertension; Ewing sarcoma, which may secrete vasopressin; insulinoma, which presents with hypoglycemia; and adrenal or gonadal tumours, which secrete steroids. None is common.

Secondary effects

The natural (and usually proper) instinct when a tumour has been diagnosed is to treat it. In the context of intracranial neoplasms, it is worth making the point that surgery and/or radiotherapy must make the endocrine situation worse, unless the treatment is directed at effecting an endocrine cure, such as the removal of a pituitary adenoma for the cure of Cushing disease. Indications for treatment of, say, a craniopharyngioma or hamartoma should therefore be on neurological not endocrinological grounds. If endocrine treatments are needed because of the position of the original tumour, they are likely to become more complex after its surgical treatment.

Surgery

The presence of a tumour sited away from the hypothalamo-pituitary area has effects on GH pulsatility, and these are increased by surgery alone and exacerbated by radiotherapy. A lesion around the area of the hypothalamus and third ventricle may cause symptoms and signs of raised intracranial pressure and may also directly affect the hypothalamo-pituitary-target gland axes (Fig. 9.1) either by affecting the release of hypothalamic hormones or by preventing their delivery to the pituitary gland. Such a lesion may present with diabetes insipidus, gonadotrophin, ACTH or GH deficiency or tertiary hypothyroidism. The replacement of cortisol may unmask latent partial diabetes insipidus. A pituitary lesion may affect the secretion of pituitary hormones directly either to increase or decrease them with appropriate clinical consequences.

After surgery in this area, any or all of the hormones may be affected.

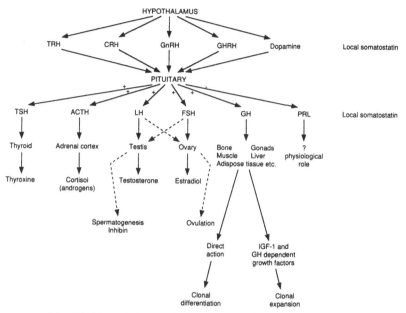

Fig. 9.1. Hypothalamo-pituitary–target gland axes.

Since ACTH (glucocorticoid) deficiency is the only life-threatening problem, all patients undergoing surgery to the hypothalamo-pituitary area should have steroid cover. Often this is administered by the neurosurgeon as dexamethasone to reduce surgical edema but, if not, it should be supplied as a pure glucocorticoid, such as prednisolone at a rate of not less than 20 mg/m^2/24 h for the first 48 hours, reducing to half of this dose for 2 days and then reducing much more slowly to reach a maintenance dose at the end of a week. Because measurements of water balance induced by increasing or decreasing ADH secretion may be difficult to interpret, glucocorticoids which have a mineralocorticoid action when given in large amounts, such as hydrocortisone, should be avoided in the perioperative period.

In the immediate postoperative period, measures to ensure very strict fluid and electrolyte balance should be maintained. Urine output may go up or down and vasopressin (in practice DDAVP) should *never* be given unless, or until, a mismatch has been demonstrated between plasma and urinary osmolalities. It should not be administered solely on the base of urine volume, specific gravity or osmolality, however disordered these may seem to be, unless plasma values have been obtained contemporaneously. DDAVP replacement may be required only temporarily while supraoptic neuronal function recovers after pituitary surgery. If a patient has been started on DDAVP replacement in the perioperative period after demonstrating a mismatch between plasma and urinary osmolalities, it should not be assumed that this is a lifelong necessity.

Occasionally, thyroxine concentrations fall precipitately after hypothalamo-pituitary surgery due to TRH or TSH deficiency. Usually they take some weeks or months to do so but this may not always be the case. The addition of GH later may cause sufficient stress to the hypothalamo-pituitary–thyroid axis to unmask a latent insufficiency.

Gonadotrophin deficiency is particularly common after midline trauma. It should be anticipated and sought after surgery and other major trauma such as road traffic accidents so that the patient who needs to have puberty induced is not left with a prolonged delay before this complication is recognized and treatment instituted.

After surgery has been performed and any subsequent treatment (e.g.radiotherapy) completed and the patient stabilized on whatever replacement treatment has been shown to be necessary in the perioperative period, six weeks should be allowed to pass before the patient is recalled for formal assessment of long term requirements for anterior and/or posterior pituitary hormone replacement. Until the results of this assessment are available and the patient has been shown to have adequate ACTH reserve, he or she should be maintained on glucocorticoid (hydrocortisone) replacement therapy at a dose of about $15\,mg/m^2/24\,h$ given in two doses, two thirds in the morning and one third at night. DDAVP should be continued during the tests of anterior pituitary function.

While the patient is still on hydrocortisone replacement, DDAVP, which may have been started in the perioperative period, should be stopped to determine the need for ongoing replacement. This may be immediately obvious or may require the performance of a formal water deprivation test.

Radiotherapy

In general, endocrine organs, with the exception of the gonads, are rather resistant to the effects of radiotherapy. Thus adrenal carcinoma is virtually radioresistant, and very high doses of targeted irradiation have to be directed to the treatment of pituitary tumours. Long-term survival of children treated with brain tumours and leukemia, the commonest malignancies, is now frequent but only as a result of the use of high doses of radiation to large areas of tissue. The endocrine consequences of this therapy are now becoming evident.

All children whose hypothalamo-pituitary axes receive more than 18 Gy develop some degree of growth hormone insufficiency. This may not always require replacement treatment, which should be decided on the basis of age, stage of puberty, bone age, genetic determination of height and family expectation, but it should be anticipated.

Growth induced by excessive calorie intake (frequent in leukemia and in children with hypothalamic lesions) or by endogenous sex steroid secretion, especially if spontaneous puberty begins early, may mask GH insufficiency. Obesity may be helped in the former by GH replacement but delay does not have long-term consequences. In the situation of early puberty, bone age may become excessively advanced and adult height compromised if a sufficient growth spurt is not engendered by GH replacement with or without additional therapy to hold up puberty.

All children subjected to cranial irradiation therefore need ongoing growth assessment and investigation and intervention if growth velocity is inadequate for the age and/or stage of puberty. When spinal irradiation has been added to cranial irradiation, spinal growth is compromised by the exposure of the metaphyses to irradiation. Limb growth is determined primarily by GH; spinal growth requires the combination of GH and sex steroids. These differential effects result in the 'eunuchoid' body proportions of patients with late puberty.

Since leg growth ceases before spinal growth, the window of opportunity for GH treatment to improve the final height of children whose spines have been irradiated can close on the unwary. Although children will have short spines after spinal irradiation whatever happens, they can be enabled to have a normal adult height by having long legs unless their GH insufficiency goes unreplaced prepubertally because therapeutic intervention has been mistimed, usually by waiting for the patient to become short before instituting treatment.

Spinal irradiation has two other endocrine consequences. The first is the exposure of the thyroid gland to the treatment. About one quarter of children whose thyroid glands are irradiated in this way develop increased TSH concentrations with time, even though the serum thyroxine concentration does not fall below the normal range. The incidence of this problem is more than doubled by the concomitant use of chemotherapy. In all children who have had spinal irradiation blood should be drawn at 1–2 yearly intervals for the measurement of thyroxine *and* TSH concentrations.

Children with elevated TSH concentrations should be treated with thyroxine replacement to reduce the TSH concentration to normal, even if their serum thyroxine concentrations are within the normal range. This is because children who have had one cancer are at risk of a second, because irradiated tissues are more likely to undergo malignant change, and because the incidence of thyroid cancer is greater in areas of endemic cretinism when TSH concentrations are raised. Treatment should be started with thyroxine in a dose of 50 mg/m^2/24 h which should then be adjusted at 6-weekly intervals to achieve a serum TSH concentration within the normal range (not suppressed below it).

The second consequence of spinal irradiation is the exposure of (especially) the prepubertal ovary, the position of which is very variable, to scatter irradiation. This leads to primary ovarian dysfunction which is detected by elevated gonadotrophin concentrations. These should be sought in the late prepuberty of a girl who has had spinal irradiation because its management may impinge upon a GH therapeutic regimen given for the consequences of cranial irradiation.

ACTH secretion seems to be the least affected by cranial irradiation. We found it in only 5% of children receiving treatment of brain tumours not affecting the hypothalamo-pituitary area. It does, however, take longer to develop than other pituitary hormone dysfunctions, so long follow-up is required.

Total body irradiation

As might be expected, the late effects of widespread irradiation of a child undergoing bone marrow transplantation are considerable. There are some data to suggest that fractionated TBI may be less damaging than single-fraction TBI.

The effects on growth are profound, first because all the metaphyses will have been irradiated and this may limit their response to endogenous or exogenous GH. The extent of this effect has yet to be determined and it may be susceptible to the effects of an increased dose of exogenously administered GH.

The effects on GH secretion are not yet clear. We have found discrepancies between provocative GH stimulation tests and GH secretory profiles. This may have important implications for the physiology of the control of GH secretion but in practical terms, the results of provocative tests correlate well with measurement of growth velocity. All children should have growth assessment after TBI, and GH treatment should be instituted early (and in generous doses) for those who do not grow well for the reasons already defined.

TSH and gonadotrophin concentrations rise after TBI and all patients should be followed to determine the necessity for replacement treatment. Recovery of gonadal function has been reported in survivors of TBI, so the long-term position has to be established in each and every patient on an on-going basis.

The hypothalamo-pituitary-adrenal axis seems to be spared in TBI in the short term but continuing surveillance is needed because ACTH reserve declines later after cranial irradiation than any other of the hormone functions.

Chemotherapy

As has already been indicated, the effects of radiotherapy are increased by chemotherapy but chemotherapy alone may affect gonadal function either temporarily or permanently. Follow-up and repeated measurement of sex steroid and gonadotrophin and of thyroxine and TSH concentrations, are needed in children who have been exposed to chemotherapy. GH and adrenal functions seem relatively resistant to chemotherapy.

Conclusion

Surgery, radiotherapy and chemotherapy all have endocrine consequences. Follow-up of growth and development of all children treated in this way is mandatory, but prolonged survival requires that such patients need life-long follow-up. Facilities for the delivery of such care need to be developed.

10

Practical matters

Endocrine tests and their normal values

Reference to Fig. 9.1 will indicate the format to be followed in this chapter. Assays have been set up for almost all of the hormones mentioned but only some are used in routine clinical practice.

Hypothalamic hormones

Because of the discrete nature of the communication between the hypothalamus and the pituitary, and because many of the hypothalamic hormones are not made exclusively in that region, measurements of them in the systemic circulation are rarely helpful. GHRH and somatostatin, for example, are gut hormones. Assays for many of these hormones do exist but are mainly for use in those rare patients who may have tumours secreting hypothalamic hormones.

Pituitary hormones

Assays of all the pituitary hormones are common and a sampling protocol in common use for testing pituitary function is shown in Table 10.1. The administration of intravenous insulin to lower blood glucose concentration is potentially hazardous. A reliable indwelling cannula must be inserted and a physician who must not be allowed to be called away for any reason whatsoever has to remain with the child throughout the procedure. For this reason, it may be difficult safely to perform such tests in a hospital where there is also responsibility for that physician to attend an emergency or obstetric department.

If a child becomes symptomatically and biochemically hypoglycemic (blood glucose concentration < 2mmol/l), an adequate stimulus to GH

Table 10.1. *Sampling protocol for the assessment of hypothalamo-pituitary function*

Time (min)	Fluoride oxalate samples			Clotted samples					
	Glucose	GH	Cortisol	TSH	LH	FSH	Prolactin	T4	E2/ Testo
0	+	+	+	+	+	+	+	+	+
20	+	+		+	+	+	+		
30	+	+	+						
60	+	+	+	+	+	+	+		
90	+	+	+						
120	+	+	+						

After Time 0 inject:
0.15 IU/kg soluble insulin.
(use 0.1 IU/kg soluble insulin in cases of hypopituitarism and after cranial surgery or radiotherapy, which includes total body irradiation.)
2.5 μg/kg LHRH up to a maximum dose of 100 μg.
7 μg/kg TRH up to maximum dose of 200 μg.

and ACTH secretion should have been applied and glucose should be administered *while sampling to measure hormone concentrations continues.* In such a situation (or indeed for the correction of hypoglycemia at any time), the following protocol should be followed:

1. **Give 10% dextrose 2 ml/kg (200 mg/kg) intravenously over 3 minutes.**
2. **Continue 5% dextrose infusion at 0.2 ml(10 mg)/kg/min**
3. **Maintain blood glucose concentration at 5–8 mmol/l for the remainder of the test.**
4. **At the end of the test, feed the child. If hypoglycemia has been difficult to control, give hydrocortisone 100 mg i.v. before removing the intravenous cannula.**
5. **Use glucagon only if venous access is lost (also see page 150).**

Before undertaking an assessment of hypothalamo-pituitary function, a clinician needs to be assured that the laboratory with which he collaborates takes part in an external quality control scheme. If there is an interest in collecting samples for research, the user needs to have figures for precision and bias of the assays being used. Every laboratory and clinician ought to agree on clinically relevant reference ranges.

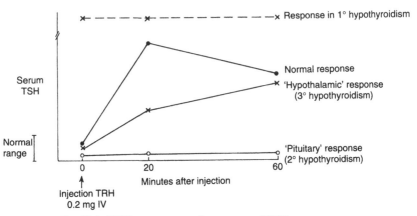

Fig. 10.1. TSH responses to intravenous TRH.

(a) *TSH* is secreted in a pulsatile fashion but spot samples do accurately reflect feedback mechanisms. If the concentration is greater than 5 mU/l, the patient probably has primary hypothyroidism (except in the neonatal period when the TSH surge may lead to levels > 50 mU/l for a few hours). If the concentration is below the limit of sensitivity of the assay, the patient probably has thyrotoxicosis. Normal levels are between 1.5 and 5 mU/l.

The administration of TRH (7 μg/kg up to a maximum dose of 200 μg intravenously) provides useful additional information (Fig. 10.1). In a normal response the basal concentration rises in a 20 minute sample and falls by 60 minutes. In primary hypothyroidism, the basal level is high and cannot rise higher; in secondary hypothyroidism the basal level is normal or low and does not change; in tertiary hypothyroidism the low or normal basal level increases at 20 minutes and is higher at 60 minutes; in thyrotoxicosis the TSH basal concentration is below normal and cannot be stimulated.

(b) *ACTH* has a circadian rhythm. Spot samples, which have to be collected, spun immediately in a cooled centrifuge and frozen, are helpful only in combination with a simultaneous measurement of plasma cortisol concentration. If cortisol concentration is < 200 nmol/l and ACTH > 100 ng/l, the patient probably has Addison disease. If the cortisol concentration is < 200 nmol/l and the ACTH undetectable, the patient probably has ACTH deficiency.

If cortisol concentration exceeds 500 nmol/l and ACTH is detected, the patient probably has Cushing syndrome. If the ACTH concentration is less than 100 ng/l, the diagnosis is probably of Cushing disease (pituitary origin); if the ACTH level is very high, an ACTH secreting tumour must be presumed. If cortisol concentration exceeds 800 nmol/l and ACTH is suppressed, an adrenal cause of Cushing syndrome can be presumed.

The administration of CRH is useful only in the assessment of pituitary-dependent Cushing disease to determine the position of an adenoma by ACTH sampling from the petrosal sinuses. This technique has not proved useful in children because of the mixing of pituitary venous blood. MR imaging is better at localization of the lesion.

(*c*) *LH* and *FSH* are usually low or absent in prepubertal children. At puberty they may be detected in spot samples up to concentrations of 10 U/l but are often undetectable because they rise only at night in a pulsatile fashion. In adult men they should not exceed 10 U/l but may be undetectable and be normal. In the follicular and luteal phases of the menstrual cycle, they will rarely exceed 10 U/l; at ovulation LH may exceed 60 U/l. Postmenopausal concentrations of both LH and FSH exceed 30 U/l.

A high concentration of LH and FSH suggests gonadal dysfunction. A low concentration cannot distinguish hypogonadotrophic hypogonadism from delayed puberty. The administration of GnRH (2.5 μg/kg up to a maximum of 100 μg intravenously) may provoke a response in both situations but absence of response does suggest the former. Repeated administration of GnRH may succeed in provoking a pituitary response in a patient with hypogonadotrophic hypogonadism; it will fail to do so in a patient with pituitary gonadotrophin deficiency.

LH may be used as human chorionic gonadotrophin (HCG) to stimulate testosterone secretion by testes in a patient of any age. There are several protocols: we favour giving 1500 units on alternate days for three injections and measuring plasma testosterone before the first injection and one week later. A normal testis will generate a testosterone concentration >9 nmol/l at any age.

(*d*) *GH* is secreted in a pulsatile fashion, so spot samples are rarely useful unless GH concentration exceeds 20 mU/l, which excludes GH insufficiency. An undetectable concentration means nothing. Because of the improbability of sampling at the time of a spontaneous peak of GH secretion, GH concentrations >50 mU/l are suggestive of gigantism or acromegaly. In a normal subject, such a high level can be suppressed to <1 mU/l by the administration of oral glucose (50 g/m^2), samples being drawn at 30 minute intervals for 150 minutes.

Tests of GH secretion (Table 10.2) should only be employed *after* a child has been demonstrated to be growing slowly. They should not be used indiscriminately in any short child.

Table 10.2. *Tests of growth hormone secretion*

Type of test	Common tests available	Comments

Screening	IGF-1
	IFG binding proteins
	Exercise
	Urinary GH
	Serum or urine collagen
	  markers
	Continuous GH withdrawal
	  sampling
		Can all detect excessively high or low levels of GH. No useful discriminant function in clinicallly doubtful cases.

Physiological	24 h profile or sleep with intermittent sampling	Complex and expensive to perform and/or analyse results.
Pharmacological	Insulin-induced hypoglycaemia Arginine Glucagon Glucose L Dopa Clonidine Prostaglandin E_2 Bombesin Galanin GHRH	Wide within, and between, subject variability. All stimuli test readily releasable pool of GH (except possibly high dose GHRH) so high false positive and negative results depending on cut-off values. Best sensitivity in detecting true positive and specificity in excluding true negative not more than 80%.

Screening tests help if the clinical situation is obvious but they fail to do so when it is not. 12 or 24 h profiles of GH secretion are time consuming and expensive and their interpretation is difficult. They are a research procedure. 24 h urinary GH secretion varies from day to day and from child to child and has not proved helpful in diagnosis.

There are many pharmacological stimuli to GH secretion and none is 100% reliable in provoking GH secretion from a normal subject on every occasion because if a test is performed just after there has been a spontaneous discharge of the readily releasable pool of pituitary GH, no further release can be anticipated. The interpretation of tests for GH secretion is difficult, especially in the peripubertal years, and since any child given GH will grow more quickly, they are not helpful in determining who should and who should not get treatment. They are best left to specialist centres.

If they are performed, any single concentration which exceeds 20 mU/l after whatever stimulus is chosen excludes GH insufficiency. Levels less than this may be seen in association with many other paediatric diseases which are associated with a low growth velocity (e.g.celiac disease), so the failure to secrete GH cannot be regarded as a specific diagnosis on a test result alone.

(*e*) *Prolactin* concentrations are very useful. A basal concentration which exceeds 400 mU/l on more than one occasion in an unstressed sample suggests a functional disconnection between the hypothalamus and pituitary and imaging is needed. A level > 1000 mU/l suggests a pituitary tumour (prolactinoma). A level < 100 mU/l and not rising in response to TRH and/or hypoglycemia suggests a pituitary lesion, which requires imaging.

Thyroid function

Basal total thyroxine concentration is the standard measurement. The normal range is 50–150nmol/l (and up to 200nmol/l in neonates). Simultaneous values of TSH should be 1.5–5 mU/l. If the total T4 is either low or high, TSH measurement should delineate the cause (see above) with or without TRH amplification. With a sensitive TSH assay it should not be necessary in usual circumstances to need other measurements.

Total T3 (1.2 – 3.1 nmol/l), free T3 (3–9 pmol/l), free T4 (8–26pmol/l) and thyroxine binding globulin (TBG, 10–30 ng/l) measurements may occasionally further illumine a thyroid problem. All other tests are obsolescent.

Adrenal function

Because of the pulsatile nature of ACTH secretion and its diurnal variation, basal concentrations of serum cortisol are not helpful for the assessment of glucocorticoid function unless they are very high (> 600 mmol/l) or very low (< 100 mmol/l), in which cases simultaneous measurement of plasma ACTH concentration is required (see above).

For an assessment of cortisol secretion, a 4-hourly profile for 24 hours is useful: in cases of suspected Cushing syndrome, we sample every 20 minutes for one hour on either side of midnight and 8 am.

24 h urine collections for the measurement of urinary free cortisol are helpful only in florid cases of Cushing syndrome: in borderline circumstances the plasma cortisol does not sufficiently frequently exceed

cortisol binding capability in children to produce a clear cut result. High resolution chromatographic separation and measurement of excreted cortisol metabolites is helpful in the diagnosis of mild cases.

For the assessment of adrenal reserve, the cortisol response to insulin induced hypoglycemia (Table 10.1) is the best test. The use of metyrapone (inhibitor of 11β-hydroxylase) with measurement of urinary steroids is not advised for children on grounds of safety. A standard dose of Synacthen (250 μg/1.73m^2) will evoke a cortisol response from any child with intact adrenal glands; a physiological dose (500 ng/1.73m^2, one five-hundredth of the pharmacological stimulus) with measurement of cortisol rise over 30 minutes can detect minor degrees of adrenal suppression.

Mineralocorticoid function is best assessed by a simultaneous measurement of plasma renin activity and plasma aldosterone concentration. Normal ranges of values depend on the assays used: ask the laboratory for their reference ranges but remember that PRA values are higher in children and much higher in neonates than in adult subjects.

Measurements of adrenal steroid precursors, such as 17α hydroxy-progesterone, and of adrenal androgens (DHAS, androstenedione, 11β-hydroxyandrostenedione) are needed for the diagnosis of adrenal steroid biosynthetic defects and a laboratory capable of measuring them should have its own reference ranges. It is not adequate to glean reference values from the literature and apply the results of an unvalidated assay to them.

Salivary steroid assays have their proponents. The values obtained have the advantage of representing free hormone concentrations but the disadvantages of spot samples.

Gonadal steroids

Plasma testosterone rises in response to nocturnal pulsatile LH secretion. Values taken in the day are low in normal adult men (but usually > 9 nmol/l) and are usually undetectable in children until late puberty. They are not helpful in the assessment of pubertal stage, clinical assessment of androgen secretion being the gold standard.

The same applies to measurements of estradiol and other estrogens in children, even if an appropriately targeted assay is used. Most estradiol assays are designed for use in measuring samples taken from adult women and levels of estradiol seen in childhood and early puberty (< 100 pmol/l) are below the level of useful function of the assay. Clinical assessment and pelvic ultrasonographic measurement of uterine dimensions are more helpful.

IGF 1 and IGF binding proteins

The measurement of these can reflect GH secretion but are not as relevant as the measurement of growth velocity (see Table 10.2). IGF-BP3 is GH dependent, but IGF-1 and the other IGF-binding proteins are also regulated by nutritional status.

Measurements of mineralization

See Chapter 7, page 130. In hypoparathyroid states, remember to measure serum magnesium concentration: in hypomagnesemic states, PTH cannot be released even if it can be secreted.

Antibodies

In any family where there is autoimmune disease, an autoantibody screen (islet cells, thyroid, adrenal) should be performed on all first-degree relatives with appropriate other endocrine tests as suggested by the results.

Imaging

Skeletal maturity

The radiographic appearances of the epiphyseal centres of the hand and wrist are commonly used to estimate bone age, an acceptable measurement of maturity because values are the same in all adults. (Such is not the case for height, weight or other anthropometric measurements so height age, weight age etc are not helpful quantities.) There are two systems of rating in common use, the Greulich and Pyle atlas coupled with the height prediction tables of Bayley and Pinneau, and the Tanner–Whitehouse system of assessment of skeletal maturity and prediction of adult height.

It does not matter which system is used, as long as it is used as its authors intended, that is rating each centre in turn and calculating the final result. The Greulich and Pyle/Bayley and Pinneau system is more robust for use in pathological cases but more easily abused by scanning the whole radiograph and applying the nearest whole standard. Bone age assessments presented with reports like 'the bone age is closest to the standard of 8 years and 10 months' are useless and so are height predictions made independently of the clinical problem. Unless a strict collaboration is maintained with a single radiologist, the clinician should learn to do bone age assessment which is very easy to learn and very quick to employ.

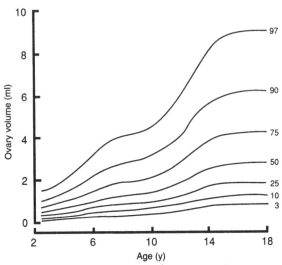

Fig. 10.2. Standards for Ovarian volume measured by ultrasound. (Kindly contributed by N A Bridges and M J R Healy.)

The appearance of the iliac apophyses can be related to the maturity of spinal growth.

Skeletal radiographs

Plain skull X-rays and coned views of the pituitary fossa have largely been superseded by CT scanning and MR imaging. Still, the majority of craniopharyngiomata calcify, and raised intracranial pressure has obvious radiological hallmarks so plain X rays should not be dismissed.

The appearances of the metaphyses in the hands and knees are valuable to assess rachitic changes.

The diagnosis of skeletal dysplasias is highly technical, and few radiologists have either the experience or interest to diagnose other than the commonest conditions. The diagnosis most frequently overlooked by clinicians and radiologists alike is hypochondroplasia. The reasons for this are twofold: clinicians may not be aware that body proportions are normal until the legs fail to grow at puberty, so only the parent(s) of an affected child may have disproportionate short stature. They may be normal, the child having a new mutation. Radiologists may not be aware that the only feature present in 100 % of cases is the failure of the lumbar vertebral interpedicular distance to widen from L1 to L5 and may not ask for the relevant AP view of the lumbosacral spine to be taken in a skeletal survey for the diagnosis of bone dysplasias.

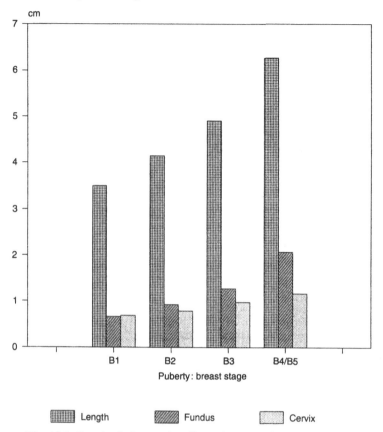

Fig. 10.3. Standards for uterine dimensions at different pubertal stages measured by ultrasound. (Kindly contributed by N A Bridges and M J R Healy.)

Complex imaging Computerized tomography (CT) and magnetic resonance (MR)

For the head, MR imaging is superior to CT. It is not clear where the balance lies between dynamic high resolution CT scanning and MR in the rest of the body.

Ultrasound

Pelvic ultrasound is invaluable for the diagnosis and management of disorders of sexual differentiation and of puberty. The results are directly related to the skill, experience and perseverance of the ultrasonographer. The technique is time-consuming, and cannot readily be accommodated beside the routine load of obstetrics and gynaecology. Reference ranges for ovarian and uterine dimensions are shown in Figs. 10.2 and 10.3.

Ultrasound is also used in identifying adrenal size and adrenal masses but it does not give results as useful clinically as CT.

Radioactive isotopes

The use of these in paediatric endocrine practice is confined largely to the diagnosis of thyroid lumps and the treatment of thyrotoxicosis. It is not necessary to scan the neck of infants diagnosed with congenital hypothyroidism since the findings will not alter management.

Bone densitometry

Dual photon absorptiometry of the lumbar spine is not recommended in children because it measures spinal height very expensively. Bone density measurements at the femoral neck and wrist are becoming of increasing interest but are not yet routine in clinical practice.

Commonly used drugs and their doses

Hypothalamic hormones
TRH

7 μg/kg up to a maximum dose of 200 μg i.v. for diagnostic purposes

GnRH

2.5 μg/kg up to a maximum dose of 100 μg i.v. for diagnostic use, less than one-tenth of that dose for therapy. GnRH therapy is rarely indicated in children.

GnRH analogues

These drugs, given intranasally, subcutaneously or, more practically, by depot subcutaneous injection (goserilin or leuprorelin acetate) are highly effective in ablating gonadotrophin pulsatility and arresting puberty. Treatment is administered monthly or, sometimes in girls, three weekly and monitored by clinical effect.

GHRH

10 ng/kg i.v. is used for diagnostic use. Therapeutic use is possible using continuous GHRH but not yet available.

Somatostatin

Native *somatostatin* and its long-acting analogue may be used in the emergency treatment of hyperinsulinemic hypoglycemia but, for suppressing GH secretion, the somatostatin analogue *octreotide* is more appropriate. The indications for the use of this agent in paediatric practice are not yet defined.

Pituitary hormones
ACTH

500 ng/1.73 m² for diagnostic purposes. Not used therapeutically because of androgen stimulation.

LH

Used as human chorionic gonadotrophin (HCG) for diagnostic purposes (see above). Used in induction of male puberty in a dose of 1000–1500 units once or twice weekly. FSH is not used in paediatric practice.

GH

The dose of *GH* used in therapy depends upon the pre-treatment growth rate, the condition being treated and the response required (see Fig. 2.11). In general, hypopituitary children require 15 units/m²/week given by daily divided injections subcutaneously. Doses of 20 units/m²/week are needed for children growing at a normal pretreatment rate and 30–40 units/m²/week for those with abnormal skeletons.

Response to GH should be monitored by growth assessment. If the response is not as predicted, the most probable reason is non-compliance with the therapeutic regimen (which applies to 40% of the patients in our clinic); a second reason is a mistaken diagnosis, of which a missed skeletal dysplasia (including the skeletal dysplasia of the Turner syndrome) is the most probable. Antibody formation is very unusual (suggesting gene deletion) as is growth hormone resistance (pseudohyposomatotropinemia).

Posterior pituitary deficiency should be replaced with *DDAVP* given intranasally at least once, and usually twice, daily. The dose at first should be 0.05 ml and increased until sufficient antidiuresis has been obtained. Serum osmolality should be checked to avoid water intoxication. Cortisol sufficiency should be assured before administering DDAVP.

Thyroid hormones

The dose for *thyroxine* replacement is 100 $\mu g/m^2/24$ h given orally as a single daily dose. The practice of giving a larger dose one day and a smaller the next is not appropriate to thyroid physiology. The dose can be monitored by growth assessment and compliance by the measurement of serum TSH concentration. Where T4 levels are normal and TSH increased, intermittent medication is much more probable than resistance to thyroid hormone action (Refetoff syndrome). Free T4 levels may also be used to monitor dose.

Some authorities recommend commencing the treatment of hypo-thyroidism, particularly in the newborn period, with *tri-iodothyronone* in a dose of 20 $\mu g/m^2/24$ h given in a divided dose three times daily. This is not usual or necessary in paediatric practice.

In cases of secondary hypothyroidism or severe myxedema, it is wise to cover the start of treatment with a replacement dose of cortisol, reducing this over two weeks.

Antithyroid medication can be given as *carbimazole* or *propylthiouracil*. For reasons not known to me the former is favoured in Europe, and the latter in USA. Rashes are common with carbimazole; agranulocytosis is a very rare complication. Medication (carbimazole 20 $mg/m^2/24$ h, propyl-thiouracil 200 $mg/m^2/24$ h) is traditionally given thrice daily initially reducing to twice or once daily and titrated against the level of serum T3 and TSH. Thyroxine may be given in combination ('block-replacement'); propranolol may be added to relieve symptoms, especially in emergency and in the newborn. In an euthyroid patient, it is not necessary to give iodine before thyroidectomy.

Adrenal steroids

Glucocorticoid replacement should be with *hydrocortisone*. The dose needed for congenital adrenal hyperplasia is rarely far from 20 $mg/m^2/24$ h which can be monitored by growth assessment. For children with Addison disease or hypopituitarism, where ACTH suppression is not an issue, a dose of 15 $mg/m^2/24$ h can be used. There is no place for using *cortisone acetate*, which is inactive, unless supply of hydrocortisone is a problem. In such instances the equivalent suppressive dose is 40 $mg/m^2/24$ h. Cortisol (hydrocortisone) needs to be given three times daily until the age of 2 years and then twice daily with two thirds of the dose given in the morning and one third at night.

Occasionally *prednisolone* is required for a more prolonged action (usually to prevent nocturnal hypoglycemia) or because it has no mineralocorticoid action; the equivalent dose is 6 mg/m²/24 h. *Dexamethasone* is suppressive of ACTH in normal subjects in a dose of 0.3 mg/m²/24 h.

Mineralocorticoid replacement should be with 9α-fluorocortisol given as Fludrocortisone acetate (Florinef®, Squibb) in a single dose of 150 µg/m²/24 h usually in the morning. Because of its glucocorticoid action (akin to dexamethasone), it is sometimes given at night to prevent hypoglycemia. Adequacy of replacement can be checked by measuring plasma renin activity; blood pressure should be monitored.

Sex hormones

Estradiol may be given orally as ethinyl estradiol, estradiol valerate or conjugated estrogens. It can be given unopposed for up to two years around puberty (and probably for longer safely in very low doses before puberty in agonadal girls) but should then be combined with a progestagen in girls with a uterus to provoke withdrawal bleeding.

An initial dose of *ethinyl estradiol* in a prepubertal girl should be 2 µg/24 h, increasing at not more than six monthly intervals to 5, 10, 15, 20 and 30 µg/24 h. Higher doses of ethinyl estradiol are contraindicated. Blood pressure should be monitored on therapy. Starting doses of estradiol valerate and transdermal estrogen are not clear.

A progestagen should be added at 10 or 15 µg of ethinyl estradiol. Suitable preparations are *levonorgestrel* (30 µg) or *norethisterone* (5 mg) given for 7–10 days every 28 days to precipitate vaginal bleeding for about 3 days.

In UK, ethinyl estradiol (20 µg) can be conveniently combined with a progestagen (Desogestrel 150 µg) in an oral contraceptive marketed as Mercilon® (Organon). The prescriber should be sensitive to the irony of prescribing a contraceptive to an infertile patient who may prefer putting up with the inconvenience of two medications. Likewise ethinyl estradiol (30 µg) can be usefully combined with desogestrel in Marvelon® (Organon) or with gestodene (75 µg) in Femodene® (Schering).

For patients without a uterus, a progestagen is contraindicated. Such patients may be treated as above with ethinyl estradiol but some physicians prefer final replacement with conjugated estrogens 625 µg (e.g. Premarin®, Wyeth).

Testosterone may be given as testosterone undecanoate 40 mg up to three times daily orally (Restandol®, Organon) but this is not very successful clinically in inducing puberty in agonadal boys. It is effective given once daily, or even on alternate days, to induce pubic hair growth in girls with ACTH deficiency.

A mixture of testosterone esters given by intramuscular injection (Sustanon®, Organon) is a reliable treatment for inducing puberty in boys. It is usual to start with 50 mg monthly increasing to 100 mg monthly, 250 mg six-weekly, then monthly, then at three-week and finally at two-week intervals spending a minimum of three and probably a maximum of six months on any dose until final replacement is reached.

Testosterone or estrogen in low doses may be used to trigger a growth spurt early in the sequence of pubertal maturation in a patient with delayed puberty. Most such patients are male and an alternative approach is to use *anabolic steroids*. Oxandrolone, fluoxymesterone or stanozolol have all been used for this purpose. Doses should not exceed 2.5 mg and a course of treatment should not last longer than six months, usually three months.

Antiestrogens are not needed in paediatric practice but the anti-androgen, *cyproterone acetate*, which also has a progestagenic action, is used both for the control of the androgen effects of polycystic ovarian syndrome (acne and hirsutism) and also for precocious puberty, reflecting its two modes of action. For the former indication, cyproterone acetate 50 mg is given daily for days 1–15 of a four week cycle with ethinyl estradiol 30 μg for days 5–26 for three months. The dose is then lowered to 25 mg given as above for three months after which an oral contraceptive should control symptoms. For precocious puberty, the dose is 100 mg/m^2/24 h given orally in two divided doses. This dose may cause ACTH suppression. A smaller dose may be used during the initiation of GnRH analogue therapy to prevent estrogen withdrawal bleeding during the initial stimulation of the ovary with GnRH.

Vitamin D

Vitamin D may be given as ergocalciferol, alfacalcidol (1α-hydroxy-cholecalciferol) or calcitriol (1,25-dihydroxycholecalciferol).

Appendix 1: SI Conversion table

	SI→Traditional	Traditional→SI
ACTH	pmol/l × 4.54→pg/ml	pg/ml × 0.22→pmol/l
Aldosterone	pmol/l × 0.036→ng/dl	ng/dl × 27.74→pmol/l
Androstenedione	nmol/l × 0.29→μg/l	μg/l × 3.49→nmol/l
Calcium	mmol/l × 4.0→mg/dl	mg/dl × 0.25→mmol/l
Cholesterol	mmol/l × 38.67→mg/dl	mg/dl × 0.026→mmol/l
Cortisol	nmol/l × 0.036→μg/dl	μg/dl × 27.59→nmol/l
Urinary-free cortisol	nmol/24 h × 0.36→μg/24 h	μg/24 h × 2.76→nmol/24 h
DHEAS	μmol/l × 368.5→ng/ml	ng/ml × 0.003→μmol/l
Estradiol	pmol/l × 0.27→pg/ml	pg/ml × 3.67→pmol/l
FSH/LH	U/l × 1→mIU/ml	mIU/ml × 1→U/l
GH	mU/l × 0.5→ng/ml	ng/ml × 2→mU/l
Glucose	mmol/l × 18.0→mg/dl	mg/dl × 0.055→mmol/l
17α-hydroxy-progesterone	nmol/l × 0.33→μg/l	μg/l × 3.03→nmol/l
Insulin	pmol/l × 0.14→mU/l	mU/l × 7.17→pmol/l
Magnesium	mmol/l × 24.3→mg/dl	mg/dl × 0.411→mmol/l
Phosphate	mmol/l × 3.10→mg/dl	mg/dl × 0.323→mmol/l
Progesterone	nmol/l × 0.31→ng/ml	ng/ml × 3.18→nmol/l
Prolactin	mU/l × 0.03→ng/ml	ng/ml × 30.0→mU/l
Renin	pmol/ml/h × 1.30→ng/ml/h	ng/ml/h × 0.77→pmol/ml/h
Testosterone	nmol/l × 0.29→ng/ml	ng/ml × 3.47→nmol/l
Thyroxine (T4)	nmol/l × 0.08→μg/dl	μg/dl × 12.87→nmol/l
Triiodothyronine (T3)	nmol/l × 65.1→ng/dl	ng/dl × 0.015→nmol/l
TSH	mU/l × 1→μU/ml	μU/ml × 1→mU/l
Vitamin D		
Cholecalciferol	nmol/l × 0.38→ng/ml	ng/ml × 2.60→nmol/l
25α-hydroxy-cholecalciferol	nmol/l × 0.40→ng/ml	ng/ml × 2.50→nmol/l

Bibliography

Essential books

Buckler JMH. (1979) *A reference manual of growth and development*. Oxford: Blackwell Scientific Publications. Contains all the growth charts needed.

Greulich WW & Pyle SI. (1959) *Radiographic atlas of skeletal development of hand and wrist*. Stanford University Press.

or

Tanner JM, Whitehouse RH, Marshall WA, Healy MJR & Goldstein H. *Assessment of skeletal maturity and prediction of adult height*. London Academic Press.

Recommended texts for further reading

Brook, CGD (ed.) (1989). *Clinical paediatric endocrinology*. 2nd ed. Blackwell Scientific Publications, Oxford. 3rd edn. in preparation for publication 1994.

Wilson JD and Foster DW (eds.) (1992). *Williams textbook of endocrinology* WB Saunders, Philadelphia. 8th edn.

or

DeGroot LJ, (ed.) (1989). *Endocrinology*. WB Saunders, Philadelphia. 2nd edn. in preparation.

Smith DW (ed.) (1982). *Recognizable patterns of human malformation* WB Saunders, Philadelphia. 3rd edn.

or

Bergsma D (ed.) (1979). *Birth defects compendium*. Macmillan Press, London. 2nd ed.

Bailey JA (1973). *Disproportionate short stature* WB Saunders, Philadelphia.

or

Bergsma, D (ed.) (1974). *Skeletal dysplasias*. Excerpta Medica, Amsterdam.

Index

Page numbers in *italics* indicate tables or figures.